'Psychoanalyst and researcher Dana Amir's book *Psychoanalysis as Radical Hospitality* is another layer in her groundbreaking thinking on the interface between language and the human psyche. The book describes in an extraordinary way deep and complex clinical material and human phenomena, extracting original and crystal-clear insights, which in combination with the wide cultural range on which Amir relies and her poetic articulation–presents a unique, exciting, and cautionary reading of mental-linguistic psychopathology.'

Prof. Merav Roth, *psychoanalyst and cultural researcher, the Israeli Psychoanalytic Society; University of Haifa; Former chair of the psychoanalytic psychotherapy program, Tel-Aviv University*

'The present book fits well with the central principle in Amir's thought. In the unique psychoanalytic type that she developed, which can be called "scientific-poetic," she examines what enables psychic movement versus what blocks, fetters, and limits it. Hence the main goal of the psychoanalytic treatment: enable the creation of a space where broad waves exist over large surfaces of sound and rhythm, rich in possibilities and meanings.'

Prof. Aner Govrin, *Tel-Aviv Institute for Contemporary Psychoanalysis; Bar-Ilan University*

'Dana Amir brings together music, poetry and photography, inter alia to psychoanalysis to deepen what I would like to think of as the "lyrical school of psychoanalysis."'

Nilofer Kaul, PhD, *Indian Psychoanalytic Society, Delhi, India;* The American Journal of Psychoanalysis, *2023*

T0372897

Psychoanalysis as Radical Hospitality

This book focuses on different forms of turning-to versus turning-away from speech across a range of experiences in clinical treatment and general life.

The chapters of this volume deal with the entrapment involved in exile from mother tongue, the parasitic language that uses the other's language as a linguistic prosthesis, the language of blank mourning which separates the mourner from their mourning, the adhesive identification of the voice and the psychotic split between voice and meaning, the mental hypotonia associated with an internalized object that turns away, and the spectrum between revenge and forgiveness. Each chapter sheds light on a different angle of the psyche's ability to spot its own leverage point and use it to transcend the infinite varieties of helpless victimhood: from the position of the victim to the position of the witness, from being the object of the narrative to being its subject, and from the position of righteousness to the willingness to forgive and be forgiven.

This book is a must read for psychoanalysts, psychotherapists and literary scholars, as well as philosophers of language and of the mind.

Dana Amir is a clinical psychologist, supervising and training analyst at the Israel psychoanalytic society, professor, vice dean for research and head of the interdisciplinary doctoral program in psychoanalysis at Haifa University, editor in chief of Maarag–the Israel Annual of Psychoanalysis, poetess and literature researcher. She is the author of six poetry books, three memoirs in prose and four psychoanalytic non-fiction books. She is the winner of many literary as well as academic prizes, including five international psychoanalytic awards.

Psychoanalysis in a New Key Book Series
Donnel Stern
Series Editor

When music is played in a new key, the melody does not change, but the notes that make up the composition do: change in the context of continuity, continuity that perseveres through change. Psychoanalysis in a New Key publishes books that share the aims psychoanalysts have always had, but that approach them differently. The books in the series are not expected to advance any particular theoretical agenda, although to this date most have been written by analysts from the Interpersonal and Relational orientations.

The most important contribution of a psychoanalytic book is the communication of something that nudges the reader's grasp of clinical theory and practice in an unexpected direction. Psychoanalysis in a New Key creates a deliberate focus on innovative and unsettling clinical thinking. Because that kind of thinking is encouraged by exploration of the sometimes surprising contributions to psychoanalysis of ideas and findings from other fields, Psychoanalysis in a New Key particularly encourages interdisciplinary studies. Books in the series have married psychoanalysis with dissociation, trauma theory, sociology, and criminology. The series is open to the consideration of studies examining the relationship between psychoanalysis and any other field—for instance, biology, literary and art criticism, philosophy, systems theory, anthropology, and political theory.

But innovation also takes place within the boundaries of psychoanalysis, and Psychoanalysis in a New Key therefore also presents work that reformulates thought and practice without leaving the precincts of the field. Books in the series focus, for example, on the significance of personal values in psychoanalytic practice, on the complex interrelationship between the analyst's clinical work and personal life, on the consequences for the clinical situation when patient and analyst are from different cultures, and on the need for psychoanalysts to accept the degree to which they knowingly satisfy their own wishes during treatment hours, often to the patient's detriment.

A full list of all titles in this series is available at: www.routledge.com/Psychoanalysis-in-a-New-Key-Book-Series/book-series/LEAPNKBS

Psychoanalysis as Radical Hospitality

Six Perspectives on Turning-to versus Turning-Away

Dana Amir

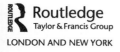

Routledge
Taylor & Francis Group

LONDON AND NEW YORK

Designed cover image: © David Wakstein: Orphanages (2014)

First published 2024
by Routledge
4 Park Square, Milton Park, Abingdon, Oxon OX14 4RN

and by Routledge
605 Third Avenue, New York, NY 10158

Routledge is an imprint of the Taylor & Francis Group, an informa business

© 2024 Dana Amir

British Library Cataloguing-in-Publication Data
A catalogue record for this book is available from the British Library

ISBN: 9781032715759 (hbk)
ISBN: 9781032715742 (pbk)
ISBN: 9781032715766 (ebk)

DOI: 10.4324/9781032715766

Typeset in Times New Roman
by Newgen Publishing UK

To Michal, Michael and Yuval

Contents

Foreword

The Archimedean Point of Hospitality

The term "Archimedean point" originates in Archimedes' famous statement: "Give me a place to stand and I will move the earth." What Archimedes had in mind was the physical point of leverage from which he would be able to lift any object, including the globe itself. The present book deals with the psyche's ability to spot its own leverage point and use it to transcend the infinite varieties of helpless victimhood: from the position of the victim to the position of the witness, from being the object of the narrative to being its subject, and from the position of the plaintiff of righteousness to a willingness to forgive and be forgiven. This transcendence implies a unique, radical form of hospitality. Although the thread woven between all these chapters is the thread of hospitality–the word "hospitality" itself is not always explicitly present in them. Hospitality, rather than being the topic or subject of these reflections, serves as their platform. In fact, one can think of hospitality as the Archimedean point that enables all these types of transcendence discussed throughout the various chapters, and therefore it also serves as the Archimedean point from which this book emerged from its very beginning: a point of departure that perceives the human being as a "lyrical whole", one who has the freedom and power to turn-to internal as well as external reality, and to raise oneself, by one's own force, from every abyss.

Acknowledgements

Every effort has been made to contact the copyright holders for their permission to reprint selections of this book. The publishers would be grateful to hear from any copyright holder who is not here acknowledged, and we will undertake to rectify any errors or omissions in future editions of this book.

The following chapters were previously published as follows:

Chapter 1:
Amir D. (2019). "Language in Exile, Exile in Language". In: Ataria Y., Kravitz A., Pitcovski E. (eds.) *Jean Améry*. Palgrave Macmillan, Cham, pp. 159–169.

Chapter 2:
Amir, D. (2020). "Parasitic Language". *Psychoanalytic Quarterly*, LXXXIX (3), pp: 527–547.

Chapter 3:
Amir, D. (2020). "The Bereaved Survivor: Trauma Survivors and Blank Mourning". *Psychoanalytic Perspectives*, 17(1), pp. 74–83.

Chapter 4:
Amir, D. (2022). "The Experience of Voice in Analytic Listening". *American Imago*, Johns Hopkins University Press, Volume 79, Number 3, pp. 517–539.

Chapter 5:
Amir, D. (forthcoming). "From "Turning-Away" to "Turning-To": Adoption as Radical Hospitality". *Psychoanalytic Perspectives*.

Chapter 6:
Amir, D. (2023). "From Actual Evil to Possible Forgiveness: Three Positions on the Axes of Self and Other". *Psychoanalytic Perspectives*, 20(2), pp. 125–145.

Chapter 1

The Language of Exile

Reflections on Jean Améry's Essay "How Much Home Does a Person Need?"

Traumatic experiences often activate a process of psychic self-annihilation. Their toxicity creates a type of psychic holes which absorb the unbearable traumatic substances along with the subject who contains them, to the point of a total collapse of inner barriers. This collapse of barriers leaves the subject imprisoned in a territory of *negative possession* (Amir, 2012, 2019), where the traumatic contents are neither digested nor worked through. The only chance of recovery from this condition lies in the possibility of depositing the traumatic substances in another subject who cannot be annihilated by them. This is the core of bearing witness (Felman & Laub, 1992; Laub, 2005; Amir, 2012).

In his *Remnants of Auschwitz* (2002), Giorgio Agamben mentions that there are two Latin words for the English word *witness*. The first is *testis*, whose etymology points at one who puts himself in the position of the mediator or arbitrator, the third party in a conflict between two sides. The second is *superstes*: the one who having experienced something to its ultimate end–can testify to it. Based on the movement between the first and the third person of experience, the function of the inner witness (Amir, 2012) encapsulates both these meanings. It refers to the ability to shift between being a *superstes*–who has undergone the full experience–and being a *testis* who mediates between the ultimate experience and language (Amir, 2019).

Agamben (2002) writes:

To bear witness is to place oneself in one's own language in the position of those who have lost it, to establish oneself in a living language as if it were dead, or in a dead language as if it were living. […] What cannot be stated, what cannot be archived is the language in which the author succeeds in bearing witness to the incapacity to speak. In this language, a

DOI: 10.4324/9781032715766-1

language that survives the subjects who spoke it coincides with a speaker who remains beyond it.

(pp. 161–162)

Since every testimony is an intersection between "what cannot be stated" and what is actually spoken, every act of testimony is simultaneously a collapse and a formation of language: a collapse of language–since bearing witness to what cannot be testified renders testimony a meaningless event, or one that conveys "archival meaning" (ibid.) only; and a formation of language–since where language succeeds to speak not in spite of the lacuna but in its name, not beyond it but through it, it becomes a true event of testimony, one that constitutes the subject of witnessing as such. In other words, in order to render account of himself, a person has to cross the abyss and simultaneously dwell in it; he must hold, within language, the unbridgeable gap between what can be said and what, exactly in being said, is elided. Agamben argues in this context that the act of witnessing is always a struggle between the one who has a voice, yet has nothing to say, and the one who does have something to say but has no voice. The witness is an exile by definition: either from himself or from language.

The Witness' Second Exile

What happens when another exile, namely the exile from one language to another, is added to the exile that is already inherently structured into the act of witnessing? It is this type of "second exile" that is the subject of the essay "How Much Home Does a Person Need?" by Jean Améry (1980).

Améry writes:

For the exiled person who came to the new country already as an adult, penetrating the signs will be not a spontaneous but rather an intellectual act, one combined with a certain expenditure of mental effort. Only those signals that we absorbed very early, that we learned to interpret at the same time that we were gaining possession of our external world, become constitutional elements and constants of our personality. Just as one learns one's mother tongue without knowing its grammar, one experiences one's native surroundings. Mother tongue and native world grow with us, grow into us [...].

(Ibid., p. 48)

The greatest rupture for the exile involves, according to Améry, the lost sensual link to language. This is not merely an inability to grasp certain nuances in the new language, or the fact that to the exile the new language presents its surface rather than its more profound strata. It is the irreversible caesura language poses for the person in exile, one that touches on his ability to relate to himself as a continuous entity: "To live in one's homeland means that what is already known to us occurs before our eyes again and again, in slight variants", Améry writes (Ibid., p. 47). Being at home implies, in other words, an accumulation of versions of existential experience whose unconscious link produces a sequence of meaning. This meaning, moreover, is not rationally elicited from language but forms in a manner that predates any knowledge of its grammar. This is exactly the rupture Améry refers to: the necessity to acquire in an intentional and structured manner what should have been a given for the speaker prior to any act of learning; the necessity to replace the mother-tongue, the language of one's home, with a language that receives the exile in a "reserved manner", as he puts it, and for "brief formal visits" only (Ibid., p. 53).

In his article "Mourning and Melancholia" (1917), Freud draws one of his most crucial distinctions, the one between the state of mourning and the state of melancholia. His key argument in this article is that in contrast with mourning–which directs itself at a concrete loss of a concrete object–the melancholic state is one where the loss is of a more ideal kind. Here it is not necessarily the object itself that has been lost but the meaning the subject associated with it: "he knows whom he has lost but not what he has lost in him. This would suggest that melancholia is in some way related to an object-loss which is withdrawn from consciousness, in contradistinction to mourning, in which there is nothing about the loss that is unconscious." (Ibid., p. 245)

And since in contrast to mourning–which is always conscious and of a real, concrete object–melancholia is an unconscious mourning of an inner, ideal object–melancholic loss is always more extensive and comprehensive than mourning, and its implications not only extend toward the future but also hark back to the past. Coping with the loss of an internal object, a person not only confronts the loss of the future (which would be typical of the condition of mourning), but also that of the past, because melancholy paints the very past in different colors than those in which it appeared before. Freud moreover argues that melancholia, unlike mourning, does not aim at the world but at the ego: "in mourning it is the world which has become poor and empty; in melancholia it is the ego itself" (Ibid., p. 246).

In my book *On the Lyricism of the Mind* (Amir, 2016) I suggested to differentiate between mourning over an actual object and mourning over a possible (Gilead, 1999, 2003) one. While mourning–however extreme–is always over an actual object (even when it is a symbolic one), as Freud put it, melancholia relates to the loss of a possible object, i.e., to the loss of the possibility it represented. It is not the person whom one loved who was lost, but love itself that was lost as a possibility, and worse than that, love never really existed in the first place, since in the eyes of the melancholic even when it seemed to exist, it was nothing but an illusion. Often a kind of "confusion of tongues" marks the state of melancholia: while the person ostensibly mourns an actual object, he does not in fact distinguish between the actual object (a specific loved one, a specific homeland) and the possible one (the very possibility of love, the very possibility of being at home). It is, in fact, this collapse of barriers between the actual and the possible that turns mourning into melancholia (Amir, 2016).

To revert to Améry: the loss of homeland he deplores is not the loss of the actual home but the loss of the possible one: "We, however, had not lost our country, but had to realize that it had never been ours" (1980, p. 50). Since this is not a mourning state of mind but a melancholic one, addressing the possible rather than the actual lost object, it focuses not on the specific loss of the specific country, but on the loss of the very possibility of being at home or having a homeland anywhere.

The internal experience of "being at home" is deeply linked to the capacity to bear witness. The melancholic collapse of the inner witness (Amir, 2012, 2019) is not the collapse of the capacity to bear witness to a specific actual catastrophe–but of the very possibility of being a witness to oneself. Thus, it extends itself toward the speaker, not only toward what is spoken about. Not only the possibility to lament the specific home is attacked, but the very possibility of being a lamenting (witnessing) subject.

Améry has a unique formulation for the attack on language in the melancholic state:

Instead of a "crumbling away of the mother tongue, I would rather speak of its shrinking. We moved about not only in the foreign language, but also, when we did make use of German, in the narrowing confines of a vocabulary that constantly repeated itself. By necessity, conversations with our comrades in misfortune revolved about the same topics [...]. Those who spoke with us did not supply our language with any new substance; they only mirrored our own. [...] There, in the hostile homeland, the evolution of the language took its course. Not that it was a beautiful language that emerged there, not that. But it was–along with enemy bomber, enemy action, front control station, indeed even along with all the actual Nazi slang–a language of *reality*. All developed speech is figurative, whether it tells us of a tree that defiantly stretches a bare branch toward the sky, or of the Jew who infuses Near Eastern poison into the German national body.

(1980, p. 52)

By means of these probing sentences Améry points at the catastrophic split between the language of the homeland and the language of exile. While the language of the perpetrator, the language of the homeland, continues its process of natural production, yielding new expressions and new images day by day–the language of exile, that of the victim, grows steadily reduced. Having been detached from its roots, it now resembles a plant which has been put into a pot. It stays alive but does not unfold as plentifully or deeply as it might have done had it remained attached to its patch of ground. It survives in terms of surface, but loses its deeper layers, i.e., the sources of its vitality.

Kristeva, in *Strangers to Ourselves* (1991), writes:

Bearing within oneself like a secret vault, or like a handicapped child–cherished and useless–that language of the past that withers without ever leaving you. You improve your ability with another instrument, as one expresses oneself with algebra or the violin [...]. You have a feeling that the new language is a resurrection: new skin, new sex. But the illusion bursts [...]. Thus, between two languages, your realm is silence. [...] Silence has not only been forced upon you, it is within you: a refusal to speak, a fitful sleep riven to an anguish that wants to remain mute [...]. Saying nothing, nothing needs to be said, nothing can be said. At first, it was a cold war with those of the new idiom, desired and rejecting; then the new language covered you as might a slow tide, a neap tide.

(pp. 15–16)

The language of exile, the language of the "neap tide" as Kristeva puts it, is a language that sticks to what we call "a secure mode": a limited, barren computer mode allowing for the survival of basic functions at the cost of all other, more complex ones. In this sense the caesura of exile is catastrophic: the continuation of life depends on amputation, but this amputation demands nothing less than life itself as its price. However, the traumatic rupture of language does not relate only to the exiled person's detachment from his concrete roots. It is also related to his experience of these roots as tainted, an experience which causes him to resist any contact with them: "Finally, whether we resisted or not, our mother tongue became just as inimical as the one they spoke around us" writes Améry (1980, p. 53). This is the unbearable paradox of the forced exile: though isolation from his deepest origins seems to enable his survival as a speaker, it malignantly and irreversibly impoverishes his position as a subject in and of language. Being isolated from his mother tongue leads to a situation in which all speech acts simultaneously link and attack linking (Bion, 1959), enable and disable continuity: "The hostile home was destroyed by us, and at the same time we obliterated the part of our life that was associated with it", writes Améry (1980, p. 51). Since he experiences his yearning for home and mother tongue as emotional manipulation, "journeys home with falsified papers and stolen pedigree" (Ibid.), he turns his back on it. But denying this home sickness turns out to be a denial of his own self: "He looks back–[…] and he doesn't detect himself anywhere" (ibid., p. 59). Améry can be seen to describe here two types of "alienation from the self" (ibid., p. 43): one is reflected in a type of yearning for something that apparently never belonged to him in the first place; the other is the alienation associated with his turning away from this yearning. It is between these two types of alienation that Améry finds himself dangling like between two abysses.

In *Black Sun* (1987), Kristeva proposes a fascinating distinction between "objectal depression" and "pre-objectal depression". For the one who suffers from pre-objectal depression, namely the child who never had a mother whose absence can be mourned–sadness is the only object. Taking the place of the lost (or never present) object, it becomes itself the object of attachment to which the deepest yearning goes out. Sadness, in such cases, may be understood as a defense against fragmentation, a mechanism which restores, albeit in pathological ways, the affective coherence which was lost to the self or never created. Reading Améry in Kristeva's terms enables us to think of this double alienation as the most profound lamentation about what he has lost. No longer existent as an object, the homeland language takes on the status of a "pre-object"–whose presence can only be marked or preserved through the obsessive clinging to its absence.

The Collaboration of the Exile

Towards the end of this essay, Améry mentions the poet Alfred Mombert, a fellow prisoner in the camp in southern France. Mombert concludes a letter in which he tells a friend what has befallen him, with the question: "Has anything similar ever happened to a German poet?" (1980, p. 59). Améry writes: "[…] Only someone who writes poetry not merely *in* German but also *for* Germans, upon their express wish, can be a German poet" (Ibid., p. 60). Further on he writes: "His readers of yesterday, who did not protest against his deportation, had undone his verses" (Ibid.). In order to be a German poet, it doesn't suffice just to write in German; one must supply for the needs of the German nation, that is, to satisfy the needs of the perpetrator, to identify with the aggressor's needs, in Ferenczi's (1988) terms. According to Ferenczi, a subject threatened by someone who terrorizes him will do his utmost to obey the latter's every wish and desire. This is not a mere external form of obedience, but an introjection of the aggressor, becoming one and the same with him. In this way the subject stops being himself and assumes the image of the other's desire. Writing in German, Améry argues in this context, is nothing but the introjections of the German nation and its needs into the subject's language, in fact erasing the subject himself from that language. And thus the reason why Mombert was robbed of his identity as a German poet was not only related to the German nation's silence regarding his being expelled, a silence that erased both his future and his past as a poet, as Améry observed. It was rather related to the fact that writing in German became an ambiguous act. Its being rooted in the perpetrator's language sentenced this poetry to the dubious status whereby pretending to reclaim the German language it repeats, in fact, the speaker's very expulsion from it.

The tragic paradox of the exile from language is associated with the fact that both agreeing with, and refusal of, exile–are types of collaboration with the erasure of the speaking subject. In the exile of language, or in the exile from language, what saves from death is simultaneously what threatens life. The tragic nature of this psychic territory is related to the fact that in it, the exiled is ordained to eternally pursue a past which on the one hand must not be looked at, and on the other hand will forever be the primal condition for every gaze.

References

Agamben, G. (2002). *Remnants of Auschwitz: The Witness and the Archive* (trans: D. Heller-Roazen). New York, NY: Zone Books.

Améry, J. (1980). "How much home does a man need?" In *At the Mind's Limits* (trans: Sidney Rosenfeld and Stella P. Rosenfeld). Indiana: Indiana University Press.

Amir, D. (2012). The inner witness. *International Journal of Psycho-Analysis*, 93, 879–896.

Amir, D. (2016). *On the Lyricism of the Mind: Psychoanalysis and Literature*. London & New-York: Routledge.

Amir, D. (2019). *Bearing Witness to the Witness: Four Modes of Traumatic Testimony*. London & New-York: Routledge.

Bion, W. (1959). Attacks on linking. *International Journal of Psycho-Analysis*, 40, 308–315.

Felman, S. and Laub, D. (1992). *Testimony: Crises of Witnessing in Literature, Psychoanalysis, and History*. New York, NY: Routledge.

Ferenczi, S. (1988). Confusion of tongues between adults and the child—The language of tenderness and of passion. *Contemporary Psychoanalysis*, 24, 196–206.

Freud, S. (1917). Mourning and Melancholia. *The Standard Edition of the Complete Psychological Works of Sigmund Freud, Volume XIV (1914–1916): On the History of the Psycho-Analytic Movement*. Papers on Metapsychology and Other Works, 237–258.

Gilead, A. (1999). *Saving Possibilities: A Study in Philosophical Psychology*. Amsterdam: Rodopi.

Gilead, A. (2003). How does love make the ugly beautiful? *Philosophy and Literature*, 27(2), 436–443.

Kristeva, J. (1987). *Black Sun: Depression and Melancholia* (trans: Leon S. Roudiez). New-York: Columbia University Press.

Kristeva, J. (1991). *Strangers to Ourselves* (trans: Leon S. Roudiez). Columbia: Columbia University Press.

Laub, D. (2005). Traumatic shutdown of narrative and symbolization. *Contemporary Psychoanalysis*, 41, 307–326.

Chapter 2

Parasitic Language

Yan, a single man in his late forties, entered analysis about three years ago suffering from a sense of deep despair. Though he is in a senior academic research position, he feels that his name is attached to achievements that are not really his. He has falsified and blown-up items in his professional CV, he teaches subjects about which, he believes, he has no proper knowledge; he is considered a good teacher because he manages to put up a false show of intelligence and devotion, but he feels he is a complete fake. For instance, he has several papers that became extremely popular in his research field but are, in fact, a patchwork of other people's ideas which he camouflaged and appropriated.

Yan is the only son of parents who were both Holocaust survivors. Yan describes his father, a simple worker, as weak and worthless, while his mother, who came from a very privileged family, is described as brilliant, well-educated, and aggressive. The mother kept Yan close to her in a perversely intimate manner: on the one hand she shared with him her deepest concerns and distresses; on the other hand, she repeatedly abused him. For instance, she used to stage scenes in which she would put food on the table without providing a plate for Yan. When he would ask for his plate, the mother would say: "But you have already eaten. Now it's our turn to eat, not yours. Those who are sitting here have not yet had their meal, but you have." She would leave him in tears and hungry only to give him food hours later. Scenes of this kind happened repeatedly throughout his early childhood. He cannot tell whether his mother saw them as a game, however cruel and abusive, or was rather acting on a psychotic belief that he really had had his meal, perceiving him as seeking to rob her of her own food.

Throughout his adolescence his mother spent long hours sharing her intellectual interests with him. Together they would listen to lectures,

DOI: 10.4324/9781032715766-2

concerts, quizzes. Yan remembers the big discrepancy between these intimate moments–during which he was mainly silent, listening to her putting herself into words–and moments when he dared asking something for himself or voicing his own ideas. These expressions evoked various types of contempt and humiliation.

Yan has never had a meaningful relationship with a woman, and always felt that he was unable to create or maintain such a relationship because he had nothing to offer. He frequents prostitutes and depends on their services. The kind of prostitutes whose services he uses belong to the BDSM[1] scene: they enact dominatrixes with masculine traits who humiliate him on account of his small penis. It is only with them that he can have sexual intercourse, and here too, only when he takes a position of absolute physical inferiority and in enactments of scenes in which they forcefully demand his sexuality. These staged scenes, in which Yan acts the weak, inferior one who must satisfy the dominatrixes who use him for this purpose, may be understood as parts of an artificial production of the familiar internalized scene of Yan serving the needs of the dominant primary object.

The great distress that makes him seek psychoanalysis relates to his feeling that he has absolutely no ability to realize his intellectual creative potential. While he dreams of creating his own new "theory of the universe", he has been suffering from writer's block for close to twenty years and can only recycle already existing materials (some of them, as said, not even his). He has a recurrent death wish that he cannot carry out for lack of courage. He spends most of his time lying in bed, asleep or masturbating, his mind barren and empty.

Yan has a history of about eight psychotherapies, each of which was marked by transgressions of boundaries: one therapist allowed him to spend all hours of the day in the waiting room; another agreed with his request to meet in a café rather than in his office. He remembers how quickly he learned what interested or attracted his various therapists by obsessively studying their body language, facial and linguistic expressions. He used to mechanically provide those contents, feeling loved for a moment–but then depleted, exploited, and abandoned.

Something similar is happening with his students. He has a great aptitude for pinpointing what it is they need; he satisfies those needs with pretense generosity (helping them to generate a successful scientific project or a new research idea), in fact binding them to himself, magically and illusively.

Yet in the end he comes to feel they exploited him. Time and again in such interactions, he is momentarily omnipotent, only to become drained into an experience of total impotence.[2]

One reason for turning to analysis involved a hope that the analytic setting would help him turn inward and release him, at least to an extent, from his compulsive fixation, as he describes it, on the other's desires. This, however, is exactly why he experiences analysis as a torture. Since he does not see my face, he has difficulty identifying "what I need from him", and therefore cannot figure out the crack through which he can infiltrate me. He knows no other way to be in touch: only by means of the exact identification of and catering for the other's needs. During our meetings as well as between them, he is obsessively preoccupied with me, something which I experience as troubling and persecutory.

In time, I notice syntactic structures in his speech that resemble the way I express myself. This is an elusive, subtle quality: Yan does not crudely "stick" parts of my mode of speaking onto the surface of his. Rather, he quietly infiltrates the spaces of my language, adopting with sophistication and probably unconsciously, metaphors that resonate mine, syntactic structures that are somehow reminiscent of my syntax. At the beginning this gave me a vague sense of closeness. But as his analysis goes on, this resonance causes a kind of distress, maybe even claustrophobia, as though something in this language-familiarity constrains and suffocates me. There are times in which it even causes me to unconsciously react by producing language that is alien to myself (slang, for instance, or other registers that are "lower" than my usual speech), in order to make a distinction, to differentiate, to create a space in which I can move freely. When Yan senses my withdrawal, he responds with outbursts of hate. This rarely happens in the session itself. But following a session during which he felt that I broke the bond of similarity between us, he usually brings a letter which he reads aloud to me, one in which he mocks and humiliates me, slams things I have said. Such moments tell me something about the function of these parasitical zones, which prevent contact with zones marked by hatred and envy. As long as we share the same language, he feels my thoughts are also his, namely that we share, over and beyond a language, a common "mind" which we both sustain. As soon as I put out my separateness—and in a sense demand ownership of my language and my thoughts—I expose his dependency on me and arouse his hatred. This obviously resembles the scenes he described between him and his mother, scenes in which he finds himself humiliated and scorned each time he has the temerity to claim his separateness.

In one of the sessions, he confesses that he repeatedly listens to my lectures on the Web to "fill the void." At the following session, the following exchange took place between us:

P: You know, on the way home I suddenly remembered these regular lunches with my mother. She would be telling me about her university studies. We'd be talking only about her, always about her, never about me. It would take hours, with her endlessly lecturing me on all sorts of things. Another child would have escaped right from the start. Or else he would just have stopped listening to her. But to me it was interesting. On the other hand, she really couldn't care less whether I was interested or not. She just used me as the passive audience of her never-ending performance.

A: It suddenly strikes me that when you listen again and again to my lectures on the Web, it takes you back, in a way, to those lunch times with your mother: they trigger a certain curiosity in you, on the one hand, but on the other, they also erase you, kind of "talking over your head", not quite at you, about my world rather than yours. So when you listen to them repeatedly, telling yourself that you are filling up a void, what happens is in fact the opposite: you make this void larger.

This is the double-edged sword of parasitical language: on the one hand, it fills the void of the missing self with the overarching presence of the other. On the other hand, it prevents, exactly in this way, any possibility for the self to emerge.

In another session Yan tells me:

P: After our last meeting I went on to meet a student of mine. And sure enough, I found myself in no time exploiting your insights as a powerful tool to penetrate her. The intensity was astonishing. Like I never even processed it at all, or internalized it, as if I never even understood that what you said was meant for me. I just used it like some means of survival, in order to get through to her.

A: So you used my words to get to another woman, in fact, used my words as a kind of artificial penis in order to penetrate another woman.

P: Well, that's what I have been doing all my life.

A: ?

P: Using all kinds of prosthetic organs in order to get women who wouldn't look my way otherwise. Exactly like I use other people's ideas to present myself as a promising researcher. I find a crack in the woman who's facing me, and I make my way in through it, only by stolen means. That's how it always was in my therapies, too. I was not at all busy with myself or with my therapy. Instead, I was into the attempt to break the therapist's code, to get into her. You know what's my biggest problem with you? I can't figure out what you need from me. I mean, I assume you need something from me, or else you wouldn't let me be here, but I don't get what it is. That's why I do creepy check-ups on you and watch you on the sly. You remember that I threatened, early on, that I could come here in the middle of the night and just sit down at the door? I didn't do it, and I don't suppose I will, but you know what? I regret it. I would like to be the one who imposes himself on you.

A: You don't feel you can really be invited into my inner space. The only way you can enter is either by sneaking in stealthily, or by imposing yourself on me violently. Even when that works, it feels like a failure because in your experience it's always infiltration, not a door that has been really opened for you.

[Silence]

P: I don't really snoop on you, like sneak peek into your house, you know, but I do watch you. I go to events I know you attend, without you knowing I'm there, I read every entry on you on the internet, there's this alert that comes up each time you're mentioned. I know about your family, or at least, I think I know, I check the dedications in your books against real persons–I investigate.

[Silence]

A: You're trying to find the crack through which you can penetrate. Maybe because you don't feel entitled to be curious about me in a natural way, curious like a child who wants to get to know the inner life of his mother, to get to know who she is, and in that way also to be allowed to know himself.

P: I never ever was that child. I was never "allowed" in. My mother either threw me out or forced her inner space on me. And I was never allowed to know anything else but her. Certainly not myself.

This is a good illustration of how Yan uses my language, sometimes like a band-aid to patch up the torn parts of his language (and his experience as a speaker), sometimes like a prosthetic body part by means of which he contrives a false sense of potency. Both the wish to penetrate his student and the wish to invade me are related to the fact that the only way of being is through an other whose desire Yan can colonize or occupy. The question that guides him is not "Who is he?" (Yan himself) and not even "Who am I?" (his analyst) but rather: "What do I want from him?" If only he knew what I desired from him, he could calibrate himself accordingly and exist (but also be erased) by means of this calibration. Rather than serving as an object Yan can use to know himself, I function as an object that presents itself as the one and only subject of knowledge, one that prevents any other object, especially Yan himself, from being knowable.

In Bion's (1959, 1962a, 1962b, 1970) terms, while in a functional course of development the maternal object enables the infantile subject to know her and by means of this knowledge confirms the child's freedom to be curious also about himself and the world–in the case of Yan's parasitic language the primary object presents herself as the exclusive object of knowledge: it is only this object, and this only object, that he is allowed to know. Any other knowledge is forbidden and blocked. In such conditions, the only language that has a chance to develop is one that imitates the object's language and annihilates any kind of difference or separation. While the mother conducts herself as a parasite within the child's language, this parasitic relationship, in a circular manner, also turns the child's language into a parasitic language which only exists by colonizing the mother's language spaces. In this malignant scenario thinking transforms into a "space-occupying lesion"– rather than a vital process. In it, a central object of thinking (the mother) develops metastases, thus creating secondary objects in her own image, imitating the natural development of language and thinking while actually blocking them.

Yan's adult relations are an agonizing repetition of this internal scene. For instance, he used to contact well known researchers in his field, putting himself in the role of their ghost writer, bringing to bear his impressive intellect in order to help them realize their own projects without getting any credit himself. One can of course equally think of Yan himself as a kind of parasite who uses other people's ideas in order to present to the world–if not to himself–a false manifestation of thinking and language. The trait of parasitism, as said, is spiral.

Piera Aulagnier (2001) wrote at length about what she called "the psychotic potential". Here the infant's primary environment of mother-infant relations produces an ambiguity in which the infant cannot know what he or she experiences. The mother's unconscious wish, in the case of psychotic potentiality, is not to give birth to a baby who is a subject in his own right, but rather to give birth to herself by means of this baby. In other words, the mother unconsciously wishes to offer her baby to her own mother and thus recover the pleasure of her own birth. This wish is none other than a death wish aimed at the infant: the mother's imaginary horizon for this baby is not his future, but rather her own past, to which she is trying to return. Thus, the baby is born to give the mother her childhood, not to enjoy a childhood of his own. This wish usually appears in camouflage, its concrete expressions taking the form of aggression towards the child (the dinner scene can be considered as this type of camouflaged death wish of the mother towards Yan). Aulagnier puts a lot of weight on the mother's role as the "word-bearer" who gives the infant the tools for thinking and language. The mother owns words and thoughts, and since the infant's undeveloped mind is in intensive contact with hers, it becomes saturated with them. Aulagnier sees the mother's influence on the infant's psyche as "primal violence". Any interpretation of the infant's feelings exerts certain violence as it imposes the mother's power of thinking and speaking on the infants' helpless psyche. Some primary violence is normal and even necessary for building that part of the ego which constitutes meaning. But the imposition of the mother's mind on the immature mind of the "future psychotic" is exaggerated. It demands that reality will appear and be perceived strictly as she describes and perceives it. This persistent demand eventually blocks the infant's ability to give meaning of its own to any feeling or experience. Aulagnier argues that this total control the mother exercises over the infant's thoughts involves a denial (initially hers, but it becomes the child's as well) of her death wish in relation to him. If he doesn't think what she forbids him to think, he will not know whatever she forbids him to know. In order to avoid the danger involved in any exposure of the unconscious desire for the death (or un-birth) of her child, the mother forbids it any contact with whatever may be associated with that desire.

Thus, the child's internal representation of the mother is one of an object who seeks to be born through him rather than to give birth to him. In Aulagnier's terms, one can think of Yan as struggling with a devouring internalized maternal object who seeks to appropriate his vital and creative powers. Rather than being a nurturing maternal object, it looks for sustenance through and at the expense of the child. Yan's later adult relations are cast in the same paradoxical mould, where his way of attaching himself to the other serves simultaneously as the one possible way of being–and as the manner in which his existence is constantly erased.

In this context, Laplanche's ideas tie in with Aulagnier's. According to Laplanche, a "fundamental anthropological situation" characterizes the human infant who comes into the world in a state of helplessness, a state which, under normal circumstances, is adequately made up for by the mother or her equivalent. Unless the situation is catastrophic, parental "messages" relating to basic needs are easily understood and integrated by the infant. However, there is always a surplus, an excess, a "noise" in the communication stemming from the fundamental asymmetry between the two partners, which fails to be understood and integrated harmoniously. This communicational "noise" is the mystifying presence of the adult's sexuality. This repressed sexuality is bound to contaminate the channels of communication, conveying a meaning that is enigmatic for the child as well as for the adult. This is an inevitable failure of translation which denotes a process of repression. The unconscious is made up of those inassimilable remnants, the residues of the failed translations of the other's messages. Laplanche refers to such a process, which he calls *implantation*, as the "general seduction", the inevitable result of the adult-infant interaction, considering the asymmetry between their respective psychic structures (Laplanche, 1987 [1989]; Scarfone, 2013). When it comes to the pathogenic aspects of seduction, Laplanche refers to *intromission* as opposed to *implantation*: implantation is a neurotic process which allows the individual to take things up actively, at once translating and repressing. Intromission, on the other hand, is its violent variant which puts an element resistant to all metabolization into the subject's interior (1998, p. 136). By depositing elements that are resistant to metabolization and thus fundamentally resistant to translation, intromission performs a kind of hijack, crippling the apparatus of translation itself and generating enclaves which strain the subject's psychic development (Scarfone, 2013).

Thinking about parasitic language in Laplanche's terms, the parasitic primary scene can be reframed as one of "intromission" (1998, p. 136), in which elements that are resistant to metabolization and thus fundamentally resistant to translation are deposited in the child's psyche. But in Yan's case, unlike Laplanche's claim, the elements that are resistant to metabolization do not bear on the mother's sexuality but relate, rather, to her death wish regarding her child, a wish Yan can neither know nor repress. These elements negate the process of translation which Laplanche considers developmentally crucial. They obstruct, in other words, Yan's entire process of thinking and creativity as well as his sense of selfhood. Therefore, on the one hand, he becomes an excellent translator of the mother–in fact it is only her that he is allowed to translate–yet on the other hand the mother is exactly the one object he is absolutely forbidden to translate (since to fully translate her means to get access to her denied death wish toward him, a death wish that he is forbidden to know). As a result, these death messages that escape the process of translation continue to operate on Yan from within.

Yan's case involves another critical dimension when it comes to his internal representation of the mother's non-desire or death wish toward him. Since the mother–a Holocaust survivor who spent the entire war in flight from one hiding place to another, shifting from one type of camouflage to another–was a child who never had a chance to be a child, it seems that her unconscious desire was to regain her childhood through her own son: to be reborn, via Yan, as the child she herself was never allowed to be. In order to reclaim her lost childhood, she, in a way, appropriated his. And so, the internalized primary scene is one in which the internalized maternal object casts terror on Yan's language and thinking, appropriating Yan's life and creative powers for her own sake.

The scene around the dinner table is a shocking example of the way Yan was forbidden to understand (in Aulagnier's terms) or to translate (in Laplanche's terms) what he experienced: on the one hand, the scene is ostensibly ruled by *deceit*, with the mother forcing a distortion of the child's reality check (arguing he has already eaten when he is actually starved). On the other hand, the scene exactly reveals the untranslatable *truth* of his mother's death wish towards him. This compound attack is an assault both on his ability to tell the difference between internal and external reality, as well as on his capacity to differentiate truth from falsehood (as the external falsehood in fact sustains the inner truth: the mother's false statement that the child does not deserve a meal reflects her death wish for him). In the present, this confusion between inside and outside, between truth and falsehood, is manifest in Yan's attitude towards himself: his constant sense of deceiving his students when teaching them something he doesn't know, on the one hand assigns "truthfulness" to the false knowledge he holds, while on the other hand assigns "falsehood" to the true knowledge he does own.

A Child Being Killed

Leclaire, in *A Child Being Killed* (1998), argues that in order to become a subject or to develop into a self, the child has to kill its parents' image of itself–the one they've had prior to its birth. In order to attain independence, one must, again and again, kill the fantasmatic image of oneself as one's parents implanted it:

> Psychoanalytic practice is based upon bringing to the fore the constant work of a power of death–the death of the wonderful (or terrifying) child who, from generation to generation, bears witness to parents' dreams and desires. There can be no life without killing that strange, original image in which everyone's birth is inscribed. It is an impossible but necessary murder, for there can be no life, no life of desire and creation, if we ever stop killing off the always returning "wonderful child". [...] To give it up is to die, to no longer have a reason for living. But to pretend that we can hold on to it is to condemn ourselves not to live. There is for everyone, always, a child to kill. The loss of a representation of fullness, of motion-less *jouissance* must be incessantly mourned and mourned.
>
> (Ibid., pp. 2–3)

Those who don't mourn the child might remain stuck in a limbo of hopeless waiting to become that child. Yet those who convince themselves that they have "vanquished the dictator", once and for all, remove themselves from their sources of creativity. In other words, desire and creativity depend on this endless mourning over the child we might have been–the image of the child which we have to kill over and over again in order to extract ourselves from it. Where this child dies, there the self comes into existence.

To create our selfhood, we must untether it from the terror of expect-ation exercised by those who came before us. While our parents' fantas-matic image of us is inevitable–no child comes into the world without such an anticipatory image–it equally constitutes the wall between us and our-selves, the wall we must smash in order to be ourselves.

One could say that Yan's parasitic language failed exactly at the job of killing his mother's fantasmatic image of him: the mother imagined that

Yan was herself, or the child she should have been, and Yan, rather than killing that image in order to be born as himself–obeyed the rules this image imposed on him and went on maintaining it. Later his attitude to that image became generalized and thus reflected in all his adult object relations: he transforms with utmost ease into the fantasmatic image belonging to any other with whom he comes into contact. This is his way of relating: he spots the other's image in order to become that image. In Leclaire's terms, this is a malignant, pathological mechanism of negation of subjectivity.

Perverse versus Parasitic Language

I have previously proposed to refer to the language of perversion as "chameleon language" (Amir, 2013), by means of which the perverse subject seeks to settle inside the other's spaces, or to appropriate the other in order to live on his or her account. The perverse subject's identification of the other's needs is not a true recognition of the other's internality. It is, rather, a pseudo-identification grounded in the perverse subject's ability to adopt the language traits of the other in such a way that the other cannot identify him or her as a stranger or feel invaded by them. The perverse subject's power inheres in his deceptively flexible use of language. Adopting the other's syntax, the perverse subject uses it to entrap that other and control his or her actions. The "infiltration" of the other in this case is accompanied by an unconscious or partly conscious intention to neutralize their defenses. The perverse subject is a child who survived thanks to his or her ability to decipher the other's mental map and to develop extremely subtle mechanisms of identification. This is a child who evolved pseudo-object relations with a blocked, inaccessible object, by means of the child's ability to take on roles and change them according to what they identify as the other's need, and by means of their special capacity to fill the other's inner spaces like air. Perverse syntax identifies and appropriates the mental fingerprint of the favored object and thus gets a hold on his or her mind (ibid.).

Unlike the perverse person's chameleon language, Yan's parasitic language is not based on the perverse desire to conquer the other. While perverse language is driven by the desire to dominate the chosen other and make him or her dependent, needy, emotionally tied to the perverse subject–parasitic language infiltrates the other's language as a mechanical form of survival shorn of pleasure. Yan is unable to produce any desire of his own, and the only way he can experience desire is by attaching himself to the desire of the other. But in the parasitic scene this desire itself loses any instinctual quality and turns mechanical, lacking vitality and life. While in the case of perverse chameleon language the compulsive repetition is of the *scene of conquest*–in the case of parasitic language the compulsive repetition is of the *erasure of self*. Here the repetition compulsion is related to the subject's defeat in the face of the other's power and desire, rather than to the urge to dominate that other (as in the perverse scene).

Apropos of the subtle differences between perverse and parasitic language, the above vignette, describing how Yan uses my words in order to get through to his student, is one in which both perverse and parasitic languages come together: while starting out as a perverse conquest scene in which Yan pinpoints the student's need, leveraging it in order to penetrate her, this ends as a parasitic scene of erasure. Since he uses the prosthetic organ of my language rather than his own natural language in order to achieve this penetration, he himself is erased in it as a speaking subject. This turns the apparent scene of conquest into a scene of annihilation.

Another difference between parasitic and perverse language is that unlike perverse language, which pinpoints the other's profound wishes and attaches itself to them, parasitic language nestles itself in the other's abstract structures, adhering to the intellect, to the external surfaces of language while staying disconnected from the deep core of the other as well as that of the subject him or herself. Thus, a kind of "third floor" of abstract thinking emerges, lacking any "first floor" that allows for a living contact with domains of drive and phantasy. When the primary discourse is so entirely aimed to put a wedge between experience and thought–as Aulagnier has put it–this directs the infantile subject away from any contact with the instinctual and fantasmatic domains, both in the object and in the self.

And so, Yan's highly evolved lofty words and abstract thinking are experienced as foreign adhesions. The core from which thought emanates and to which it returns is missing. This is a two-dimensional structure (Meltzer, 1975) that borrows its three-dimensionality from the other, by using him or her parasitically as constituting this missing dimension. This can be observed in the following vignette:

P: This week I had to attend some review meetings about scientific projects that my colleagues have submitted. Can you imagine? Me! I am the review committee?! I, who don't manage to get any kind of project off the ground, I who am a total dud compared to them. So, they sent me these projects and I had to write a review, and then to meet those candidates face to face. And then this person who heads the committee says that the reports I wrote were the most brilliant, profound, sharp. What he doesn't know is that I was using somebody else's templates. There's this researcher that I admire, and I simply take a ride on what she writes. It's got nothing to do with the subject matter, there's no connection between the kind of things she writes and what I wrote in those reviews. All I did was taking the mold of her writing, using her actual sentences, and inserting the stuff I wanted to say into their syntactic structures. That's the only way I could write or say anything. Now you know what a wretch I am.

A: You need the pattern of someone else's language because you don't have a language of your own, one in which you can speak.

P: That's what's so strange. It's like I have opinions of some sort, but I lack any ability to formulate them. The only way is to use her language. Only when I use her language I can think, and then put thoughts into words.

Traumatic Traces in Language

In relation to Holocaust survivors specifically, and survivors of collective trauma in general, Yolanda Gampel (1996, 2000) formulated the notion of radioactive identification and transference. The term describes how violent elements from external reality penetrate the psychic mechanism, while the individual is totally unable to defend him or herself against their influence. This radioactive identification involves unrepresentable traces which make their way into the individual. As in the case of exposure to actual radioactive radiation, here, too, traces may only erupt years after the event, in victims as well as in their offspring. Gampel suggests that one manifestation of this phenomenon is the sudden appearance of cruelty, characterized by signs of dehumanization, a cruelty untypical of the subject's usual behaviors and attitudes (ibid., p. 64). Since radioactive identifications emerge from the unconscious, they are not subject to recollection, but can only act and be enacted.

Radioactive identifications mean that the malignant materials operate ego-syntonically rather than ego-dystonically. They don't trigger a sense of inner conflict or contradiction with declared human values. They gain their destructive power from the fact that despite their factual recollection, whole parts of the traumatic past are either not represented, or else represented in a "blank" mechanical mode, as merely archival entries (Agamben, 2002), lacking any emotional connection. In the primary scene of Yan and his mother, Yan seems to have become the recycling zone of his mother's radio-active identifications. The mother, who inflicts terror on the child's thinking–repeats in that way both the narrative of her own rescue (she survived by erasing or camouflaging her identity) and the narrative of her annihilation. This complicated quality turns this mechanism of negation into a malignant tool that acts both to execute (erasing the child as an autonomous subject) and to rescue (both the mother, who in this way regains her own childhood, and Yan himself–who in his mother's psychotic inner scene features like a fugitive whose one chance of being saved is by making himself disappear).

What we encounter here is the compulsive operation of the mother's mechanisms of death and resuscitation on her child's psyche who becomes both the one who is erased in order to be saved; the one whose erasure serves as a repetition of his mother's erasure; and the one whose erasure serves to restore the mother's lost self.

After about three years of analysis, with this direction of interpretation, Yan brings a first dream (he never remembers his dreams, and most of the time he does not dream at all): in the dream, actually a nightmare, Yan gets himself locked into a freezer and cannot get out. He feels how his words congeal on his lips, and he stops being able to articulate vowels but only consonants (in Hebrew, the word for vowel is *tnua*, which also means *movement*; the word for consonant is *itsur*, literally: a *stop*). He tries to figure out a way of talking that doesn't need vowels, only to discover it's impossible. Then he wakes up.

This nightmare gets to the heart of the phenomenon of parasitic language. It is a language that does not enable psychic movement; one in which the thinking apparatus becomes a kind of freezer (which preserves the other's desire as the only object and prevents any transformation in relation to it) instead of a vital space.

In yet another nightmare Yan is trying to break through a wall, only to discover that he himself is part of that wall and thus might be destroyed with it. Over and beyond the specific contents of these emerging dreams, Yan feels he is beginning to live a psychic life for the first time. During one of our meetings he says: "When I dream, there are two things: I know I'm alive, and I know I'm telling the truth."

In his paper "On Not Being Able to Dream" (Ogden, 2003) Ogden quotes Bion (1962) who claimed that the opposite of a bad dream (a nightmare) is not a good dream but an undreamable dream, a dream that cannot be digested, remembered, or forgotten, kept secret or communicated, but can only be evacuated through psychotic fragmentation or suicide. In a different but complementary context, Grotstein (2000) divides the function of dreaming into two basic functions: "the dreamer who dreams the dream", and "the dreamer who understands the dream". Both the dreamer who dreams the dream and the dreamer who understands the dream take part in the sense of I-ness. When these two are internalized, a function develops that corresponds to the intrinsic analyst within us all. This is "the dreamer who makes the dream understandable", Joseph the dreamer, Joseph who offers necessary perspectives of truth (ibid., p. 31).

The terror inflicted on Yan throughout his childhood attacked, in Grotstein's terms, not only the possibility of being "the dreamer who dreams the dream" (since Yan was only allowed to dream his mother's dreams, not his own), but also the capacity to be "the dreamer who understands the dream" (since he was prevented from a full understanding even of his mother's "dream", the one dream he was allowed to dream). As a result, no perspective of truth was available to him.

Both object relations and analytic relationship were destructively staged by Yan according to the same compulsive rules where the other's dream turns into the sole object. The great danger, thus, was that analysis would transform into another parasitic cycle in which my analytic dream would become another terrorizing object. To prevent this, an analytic "antibody" had to be created that would operate against the parasitic compulsive recycling. The only way to create such an antibody was by means of interpreting the parasitic mechanism itself: illuminating, each time from a different angle and in a different manner, Yan's calibrating himself to my needs (or what he perceived as such) rather than to his, adopting my language structures instead of constituting his own.

This is illustrated, for example, in the following continuation of the previous vignette:

A: It's as if there's a kind of mother tongue missing.
P: It's like what you described as the "function of the inner witness" in your book. That's what I lack. I have no witnessing function. You see, I came to you because I read your chapter on the chameleon language,

but it turns out that I am here because of your chapter on the inner witness.

A: Now you're doing the same thing with my language as what you've been doing with the language of that researcher. You make your way into my linguistic patterns (chameleon language, inner witness) in order to be able to say something about yourself. But what happens is exactly what happened with her: the moment you adopt those linguistic structures, you as a thinker, you as a speaking subject, are lost. No matter how intensively I search for you–all I find is myself.

Discussion

The real danger in the analytic work with Yan lies in the illusion that accompanies any development or vitality: given the fact that every therapist's–and certainly every psychoanalyst's–big dream is a dreaming patient, the emergence of Yan-the-dreamer poses the inevitable question whether this is a case of natural dreaming, or rather one in which he illusively dreams my dreams. In contrast with the approach whereby the dream is "truth telling", the spontaneous creation of the unconscious, in Yan's case we must also face the possibility that his dreaming may be part of his effort to leech onto my desire and repeat the scene of the erasure of his subjectivity. This might issue into a tragic paradox in which signs of life and signs of death may be truly identical, and thus phenomena like dreaming, creative thinking and desire may simultaneously suggest the presence of opposite forces.

How do we work analytically in an environment whose most prominent feature is its illusory nature? When Yan says: "When I dream, I tell the truth"–does he tell the truth? Does he dream? The one way we can work with and against this illusion is by interpreting it again and again. Thus, whenever Yan brings a dream, our work should not be limited to the dream content as such, and not even to Yan's ability to dream as such, but rather to address the fact that the very dream may be designed as a gift to me, one by means of which he is simultaneously born and aborted. Relating to Yan's dreaming as merely a sign of life would be like an enactment, in the analysis, of the dinner scene in which I would be starving him while telling him that he's eating; make him believe that he's being treated while letting him fall through the analytic cracks. On the other hand, restricting myself to seeing his dreaming only as signaling death would make a no less tragic omission by disregarding the budding dreamer who is truly making his way out through the debris.

Yan represents an extreme case of parasitic language. But this extreme case allows us to consider zones of parasitic language also within regular language, where language colonizes spaces of the other's language and performs a kind of double act of resuscitation and annihilation. Being sensitive to these zones and the way in which they play themselves out in the analytic duet is so important exactly because of their typical deceptiveness, which almost inextricably ties together signs of life and signs of death. This entanglement can be faced only by the disentangling power of the soundbox of countertransference. I realized that I react differently, often in clashing ways, to materials which mobilize annihilation qualities versus materials which mobilize living and life-bearing qualities. For instance, I reacted very differently to dreams I experienced as a way of clinging to what Yan perceived as my need than to those that I felt he brought in spontaneously. This distinction cannot always be made unambiguously, but raising the question as such is critically important.

The psychoanalytic work must do the impossible here: to balance between the poles of vitality and stasis; to hold simultaneously the danger of the death trap and the recognition that one who has died so many times and yet comes back to claim his soul must be telling something real about the unsubdued force of life he is carrying.

Notes

1 Which includes a variety of erotic practices that all hinge on a controlling element.
2 In a way, when he teaches his students things that he himself doesn't know— he "implants"–at least in his unconscious phantasy–false knowledge in them which turns them into frauds like him. His rage, and the sense of exploitation and abandonment that accompany each such scene, are connected with the fact that sometimes his students really do become knowledgeable or creative in spite of the allegedly false knowledge he implanted. This leaves him depleted both of true knowledge and of the ability to implant false knowledge in others and spoil them in that way.

References

Agamben, G. (2002). *Remnants of Auschwitz: The Witness and the Archive* (trans: D. Heller-Roazen). New York, NY: Zone Books.
Amir, D. (2013). The chameleon language of perversion. *Psychoanalytic Dialogues*, *23*, 393–407.

Aulagnier, P. (2001). *The Violence of Interpretation* (trans: Alan Sheridan). London: Routledge.Bion, W.R. (1959). Attacks on linking. *International Journal of Psycho-Analysis*, 40, 308–315.

Bion, W.R. (1962a). *Learning from Experience*. New York: Basic Books.

Bion, W.R. (1962b). The psycho-analytic study of thinking. *International Journal of Psycho-Analysis*, 43, 306–310.

Bion, W.R. (1970). *Attention and Interpretation*. London: Tavistock.

Gampel, Y. (1996). The interminable uncanny. In L. Rangell and R. Moses–Hrushovsky (eds.), *Psychoanalysis at the Political Border*. Madison: International Universities Press, pp. 85–98.

Gampel, Y. (2000). Reflections on the prevalence of the uncanny in social violence. In A. Robben and O. Surez-Orozco (eds.), *Cultures Under Siege: Collective Violence and Trauma in Interdisciplinary Perspectives*. Cambridge: Cambridge University Press, pp. 48–69.

Grotstein, J.S. (2000). *Who Is the Dreamer Who Dreams the Dream?* Hillsdale, NJ: The Analytic Press.

Laplanche, J. (1987 [1989]). *New Foundations for Psychoanalysis*. Oxford: Blackwell.

Leclaire, S. (1998). *A Child is Being Killed* (trans: Marie-Claude Hays). Stanford: Stanford University Press.

Meltzer, D. (1975). Chapter IX: Dimensionality as a parameter of mental functioning: Its relation to narcissistic organization. In *Explorations in Autism: A PsychoAnalytical Study*. London: Karnac, pp. 223–238.

Ogden, T.H. (2003). On not being able to dream. *International Journal of Psychoanalysis*, 84, 17–30.

Scarfone, D. (2013). A brief introduction to the work of Jean Laplanche. *The International Journal of Psychoanalysis*, 94(3), 545–566.

Chapter 3

The Bereaved Survivor
Trauma Survivors and Blank Mourning

"Blank mourning" is a mode of mourning unique to bereaved parents (parents who have lost their children) who themselves–or their families–are Holocaust survivors. In "blank mourning," survivors of real traumatic loss suffer an inability to mourn. Tormented by the toxic combination of survivor guilt and the guilt of bereavement, a combination of which they are unaware and therefore cannot access, they are unable to create in their minds an object of mourning, an object to be mourned, and thereby are unable to connect either to their lost objects or to their own mourning selves.

In Israel, where the real or imagined survivor has always survived another, if not at the expense of an-other, the work of mourning and its implied task of witnessing are charged beyond bearing. There is a double narrative behind entire generations of Israelis whose families survived the Holocaust, families in which the survivors carry the need to atone for the deaths of those who did not survive. Regardless of the concrete circumstances of the loss, the survivor carries a permanent imaginary scene in which he or she simultaneously takes the role of the helpless victim as well as the collaborator, whose willingness to sacrifice the other has saved him or her from death. The scene of survival, in this sense, is always based on a double narrative in which one is perceived both as a victim and a perpetrator/collaborator. This double narrative has been present in the discourse–or rather the absence of discourse–of generations of survivors. These survivors' work of mourning does not merely touch on the concrete losses they have suffered but is inextricable with the awareness that their very existence is grounded on, and to considerable extent the very outcome of, these losses.

Of the guilt experienced by Holocaust survivors, Alfred Garwood (1996) writes:

DOI: 10.4324/9781032715766-3

In the face of their cumulative losses and the inescapable yet impossible choices, of the mental mechanisms available to adapt or defend against their powerlessness, self-blame and consequential guilt were almost inevitable. It is my view that 'survivor self-blame' had the initial primary and principal function of reducing the pain and anguish of intolerable powerlessness in the face of annihilation risk and overwhelming loss. Being forced to be totally passive and helpless in the face of the Holocaust was perhaps the most devastating experience for the survivor. Survivor guilt has persisted primarily because survivors are unable to grieve and mourn their losses successfully. Whenever losses are remembered, the overwhelming feelings of powerlessness and annihilation fears that were experienced at the time of the events together with the highly effective defense of self-blame are mobilized [...]. These effectively obstruct working through and thus the mourning process.

(pp. 246–247)

Garwood's main argument is that survivor guilt functions as a defense against the greater catastrophe of total powerlessness. Guilt, even where it is unconscious, presumes choice (without choice, there is no ground neither for blame nor for guilt), thus serving as a defense against the most difficult experience of having no choice. And yet, this defense mechanism comes at an impossibly high price. An extreme manifestation of this price is the complex work of mourning of bereaved survivors: bereaved parents who are themselves Holocaust survivors or their offspring, who still largely suffer from the traces of their forbears' trauma. Their own mourning for their dead children is inevitably contaminated by these earlier traumatic traces. This contamination, yoking together survivors' guilt and the guilt of bereavement, leaves a strong impact on the resulting work of mourning (or non-mourning): preventing contact with both the object of mourning (the lost object) and the subject of mourning (the mourner her–or himself), it replaces the work of mourning with mourning rituals whose fetishistic and addictive character prevent the rich, internal dialogue which the work of mourning enables and requires.

Various authors have discussed the ambiguities of victim and perpetrator in the general context of trauma, and more specifically with reference to Holocaust victims. In her book, *Memorial Candles* (1990), Dina Wardi describes how in Europe's extermination camps, Jung's theory concerning the perpetrator-victim archetype (1946, 1952) was borne out in terrifying dimensions hitherto unknown in Western culture and perhaps worldwide. For Jung, the aggressor and the victim are two aspects of the same archetype. Each human being includes a persecutee and a persecutor. Another variant of this is the notion of the "victimator" (victim and perpetrator), a term coined by Durban (2002). This combination creates a circular dynamic in which the internal perpetrator derives power from its status as victim, and vice versa. The Jewish people have been locked in generations in this conceptual emotional position of the "eternal victim," where Israel stands in for Isaac-led-to-the-altar. However, this position always includes its opposite: even as the Jewish psyche is identified with the victim, it must also contain a sense of the aggressive, hate-propelled, and war-lusting fighter, a sense it often discharges onto the "other," the "*goy*" without or within one's soul (Wardi, 1990, pp. 97–99).

In contrast to the discussion concerning the perpetrator/victim or the persecutee/persecutor dyad, what comes to my mind in the present context is a more specific synthesis of the sacrifice and the "sacrificer" (the one who sacrifices). The figure of the "sacrificer," as the Biblical episode of Abraham's sacrifice of Isaac suggests, is a hybrid including a singular variation of both aggressor and victim. Abraham, who brings Isaac to God as a holy offering, does not have to sacrifice himself, but he is asked to make a much larger sacrifice than that of his own body: that of his son. This story holds the duality of the very act of sacrifice: at one and the same time, Abraham is both sacrificing and sacrificed. Derrida, discussing Abraham and Isaac in his book, "The Gift of Death" (1995), writes: "And it is the sacrifice of both of them, it is the gift of death one makes to the other in putting oneself to death, mortifying oneself in order to make a gift of this death as a sacrificial offering to God" (Derrida, 1995, p. 69). Within the double position of the sacrificed/sacrificer, then, one is simultaneously active and passive, victim and aggressor, murderer and heir. If we take Abraham as an archetype of present-day Israel's bereaved parents, we observe that they consider themselves, simultaneously, as victims who were forced to sacrifice their children, but also as sacrificers who *chose* to sacrifice those children for the sake of the Jewish nation and the national ethos.

This doubleness of victim and victimizer, or victim and collaborator, reproduces the historic doubleness of survivor guilt: Holocaust survivors experience themselves as having survived "at the expense" of others, or at the cost of other people's deaths. The difficulty of coping with past and present traumas involves the fact that the representation of the traumatic event is tethered to the representation of the survivors' own destructive powers: not only were they bidden to live by their dead loved ones, but in the very fact of living, they bade their loved ones to die.[1] This fusion between the role of the sacrificed and the role of the sacrificer situates the whole work of mourning in a domain of emotional and moral ambiguity. How does this ambiguity affect the resulting language of mourning?

Language is first and foremost a depressive achievement, an achievement involving both the concession of that which cannot be said, and the giving up of the symbiosis with the other, acknowledging him or her as a distinct subject. Indeed, we can say that acknowledging separation is simultaneously the driving motivation to speak, as well as the condition for establishing language (Amir, 2010, 2014). "Language is simultaneously mourning made real and unending," writes Pontalis (1980, p. 252) in a similar context. The capacity to establish language is conditioned both upon the capacity for individuation and upon the ability to mourn. Indeed, establishing language enacts a similar ambivalence to that which takes place in the process of mourning, as it implies both an adherence to the object as well as the capacity to let it go and recreate it within (Amir, 2010, 2014). Every act of speech is at one and the same time an act of negation and an act of confirmation, as Kristeva puts it: "upon losing mother and relying on negation, I retrieve her as a sign, an image, a word" (Kristeva, 1987, p. 63), meaning that the possibility to create even the word "mother" is based, in a way, on the capacity to negate her: to let her go.

Green (1986) similarly suggests that the crucial moment in the development of the capacity for symbolization is when the infantile subject becomes able to "negate" the mother's presence in order to create her as the background onto which the representations he forms (including those of the mother herself) are registered. The negative hallucination of the mother (i.e., the mother who has been "negated" by the child) now turns into a framing structure, a blank screen which is requisite for the work of representation as such. For this framing structure to come into existence, the mother must first be fully present, in order to allow her child to erase her and to form the representation of her erasure. When this is possible, the mother as primary object of concrete fusion fades and re-emerges by way of an internal foundation or substrate. This erasure of the maternal object and its transformation into a framing structure produces a container in the infantile psyche, one that is not threatened in the face of difficult emotions. The void, within this negation, becomes a necessary, enabling ground, like the white page needed for words to be written. Where a mother is mentally absent, by contrast, her erasure is not possible. Here, rather than forming a frame or ground, her absence inspires terror, creating an ongoing need for concrete clinging to the concrete object. When it is impossible to bear the void, a need arises to be in constant contact and friction with sensory objects. In other words, when the functional process of erasure cannot take place, what occurs—instead of the negative hallucination of blankness that both delineates and enables thinking (the void as a screen or ground)—is the nullification of the very possibility of psychic life, and the obsessive adhesion to the concrete surface of the concrete object.

This process describing the negation of the object as a basis for the formation of verbal language, is no less apt when we look at the language of mourning: in order to create a representation of the lost object, namely, to release it from the concrete world and recreate it symbolically, this object must first be present in a non-ambivalent way. Much like the secure attachment to the mother is the condition for her erasure and her re-creation in the child's psyche, attachment to the lost object is requisite for letting go of its concrete aspects and reproducing it within. When the lost object, however, is an ambivalent object—exactly in the same way as when the mother doesn't constitute a stable presence—it is hard to the point of impossible to release it and recreate it in a symbolic way.

In the Israeli domain of bereavement, the lost object is always an ambivalent one, both because the experience of mourning includes a mixture of the above-mentioned dimensions of sacrificer and sacrificed, as well as because the Israeli reality itself—if we extend this ambivalence—is marked by an incessant confusion between the position of absolute victim (the notion of Israel as eternal victim to enemies that "rise up to destroy it") and that of the aggressor (Israel in its role of occupying state, ruling over the Palestinian population). This confusion turns the national ethos itself into an inherently ambivalent one. Thus, a "blank mourning" takes the place of the vital work of mourning: representational failure takes the form of pseudo-representation, and the language of mourning becomes a pseudo-language (Amir, 2010, 2014).

As in Green's areas of terrifying void, in the arena of blank mourning, sensory adhesion to the concrete object replaces the ability to produce a rich inner representation of this object. This is reflected in the hollow and artificial use of pseudo-symbolic structures of language, in the recourse to clichés, and in the clinging to rituals of mourning which, like clichés, do not mediate between the mourner and the lost object but rather hold it in a compulsive grip that separates between the mourner and the pain of loss.

In an article that deals with traumatic narratives, Laub (2005) argues that in the traumatic situation the traumatic loss of the good object and the libidinal ties to it releases the hitherto neutralized forces of the death instinct and intensifies the clinical manifestations of its derivatives (pp. 316–317). I would like to suggest that where mourning is mixed with guilt, we are dealing not only with the loss of the good object but also with the loss of the bereaved as a good object in his or her own eyes. This loss sets free the previously neutralized forces of the death instinct, as Laub suggests, and the only way to control them is by drawing a line between mourner and the experience of loss by means of turning the process of mourning itself into a fetishistic object that can be held and controlled.

This resembles, to some extent, the "excessive testimonial mode" which I have previously discussed in the context of testimonies of trauma survivors (Amir, 2016a, 2018, 2019). In this testimonial mode the traumatic object becomes an addictive and gratifying object, an object whose totality replaces a functional sense of being. Testimony in this case renders the traumatic memory a saturated object (Bion, 1962a,b, 1959, 1970), an object which refuses transformation and to which the obstinate adherence becomes malignant. The deceptiveness of this testimonial mode is related to its intensive linguistic characteristics: while the register of trauma opposes language, the overt manifestation of the excessive testimonial mode is not an absence of language. On the contrary: it often presents articulate and well-developed language, with a wealth of rhetorical features. But underneath the rhetorical cover, this is a pseudo-language that attacks rather than produces linking, a saturated language that under the guise of "full testimony" presents what Caruth (1996) calls "empty grammar": an attempted reconstruction of the event which in fact erases it, and thus does not allow for its subjects to undergo transformation.

Like the excessive testimonial mode, the mode of blank mourning, too, produces a false performance of mourning. In this false performance, the act of preservation comes to substitute for the work of mourning, imitating the surface of language and rituals of mourning at the expense of the possibility of creating vital contact with the lost object.

In "Mourning and Melancholia" (1917), Freud claims, as said earlier, that in contrast to mourning–which directs itself at the concrete loss of a concrete object–the melancholic state is one where the loss is of a more ideal kind. Here it is not necessarily the object itself that has been lost but the meaning the subject associated with it (p. 245). Concerning the bereaved survivor, we may take the moral ambiguity of sacrificer/sacrificed as the "what" that remains inaccessible to consciousness, even if the mourner is perfectly clear about the lost "who." And so, in a sense the state of empty, blank mourning resembles melancholia. But melancholia is attended by a turning inwards and a withdrawal, while blank mourning converts contact with the inner world into a ritual contact, sometimes of a manic nature, with the external one.

A Clinical Vignette

Yiftach lost his son a few years ago. He himself was born to parents who were children during the Holocaust, and who lost their own parents. He asks for therapeutic help because he feels unable to cope with the loss of his son, but it gradually emerges that he has no internal access to this loss. He talks about his son's death in a language that seems taken from the official albums that the Ministry of Defense publishes on Remembrance Day, trapped in a vocabulary that includes no pain, with nothing that can be touched without being strangled by cliché.

He is tortured by the thought that his son joined the army to protect him, to save him, and he is tortured no less by the way in which this attempted rescue repeats his own birth as coming to keep and pass-on the memory of his parents' parents, who died in the Holocaust. Since his son's death, he has been caught in a compulsive ritual of mourning: he neglects his health and is out of touch with his former life, going from one TV interview to the next, from one ceremony to the next, from one memorial service to another. He doesn't feel anything, and most of the time acts in a robotic, detached way. In our therapeutic encounters, he is extremely difficult to reach. He is crashing under this eternal mourning, but equally terrified of letting it go, refusing to give up the compulsive rituals because they are at one and the same time what keeps him away from the living dialogue with his son, and what allows Yiftach to cling to him.

I notice that interventions that touch on the contents of what he says (the pain of losing his son; his guilt for having failed to protect him; the ways in which this story of sacrifice relates to his family historical story of sacrificing loved ones to survive) only calls forth the barren repetition of the hermetically blocked narrative (Amir, 2016b). The only chance to pop this bubble of blank mourning, so I understand with time, is the interpretation of its very mechanism: endowing meaning and words to the manner in which he is stuck in the empty language of collective mourning, which recruits his son's death into a narrative that justifies it in terms of the national ethos, but abandons it in terms of his private story; and casting a light on the fact that he is not imprisoned in this empty collective language as a helpless victim, but rather deploys it in order to avoid the naked contact with both the loss of his son and his own self-representation as someone who collaborated with the system that led to this loss.

Returning to the previously mentioned notion of *radioactive identification and transference* (Gampel, 1996, 2000)–Gampel (2010) suggests that the survivor's personal experiences may transform in the course of the therapeutic process in order to become integrated in a collective, symbolic narrative, and thus allow the patient to forget or at least reduce the guilt of surviving. In the case of blank mourning, however, embarking on a causal, collective chronicle is a pitfall because this collective chronicle itself is one of the symptoms of blank mourning. How so? In her book, "And Who Will Remember Those Who Remember" (2019), Cohen-Fried describes two typical Israeli "languages of bereavement": "the national language" and "the mother tongue". While the former situates the dead son as part of the extended "national family" and justifies his death by appeal to the ethos of national survival, the latter rejects this appropriation by the nation and attempts to extricate the son or daughter, and the grief for them, from it. Following Cohen-Fried I would like to suggest that blank mourning is what takes place when the internalized "national language" incorporates the internalized "mother tongue," namely, when the personal, singular narrative is swallowed or overwhelmed by the collective narrative. The national language is in fact a mechanism that negates the singular work of mourning, and that comes, in many ways, to screen the private loss. The vital work of mourning requires, therefore, a type of "counter-negation," grounded in the active negation of the national language or in the resistance to the terror the national language inflicts on the mourners–both from outside and from within.

In his book, *Falling Out of Time* (2010), the author David Grossman, who lost his son in the second Lebanon war, writes a fantastical journey of mourning, a poetic voyage to where his dead son is. The protagonist of Grossman's book walks in ever-widening circles around his house and town and is joined by an ever-larger group of parents who have lost their children, too. The book narrates a journey marked not just by his encounters with those coping with bereavement, but by the need to release his child's death from the public realm in order to restore it as a private loss. In one of the most shattering moments of this book, the father offers that his dead son "live through him". This is an inverse act of sacrifice: he, who allegedly sacrificed his son, now sacrifices himself so that his son may live. While perpetuating the myth that life always comes at a price for someone else, this is also an attempt to break this horrifying order by giving back to his son the life that his death doomed his father to live. It is exactly this conversion upon which the insight at the very end of the journey touches: the understanding that the possible death of the father will not revive the son. No one bids anyone to live by dying. Death does not command life. It does not even command death.

As the father walks in circles around the town he encounters a wall. It is a wall that cannot be crossed, and as he kneels in front of it, he observes the faces of the dead within its stones. The faces move and shift within the rigid material onto which they have been stamped, as though they were growing within it. The encirclements that the father performs around the wall are somewhat reminiscent of the Biblical encirclements of the walls of Jericho. What number of cycles must the father complete around this wall that stands between him and himself, between him and his dead son, so that the petrified, rigidified grief will give way to vivid mourning? Where memory is unbearable it often escapes thought into the body spaces. Then the body becomes a vehement and vivid scene of unconscious memory. Sometimes the body preserves the feeling of the lost loved one, sometimes the body imitates the way he walked, the way she held her head, the nuances of his or her voice. The body may imitate the illness, or alternatively mark the spot of the traumatic injury. There is an infinity of ways in which the body conserves what the mind has lost, and all these forms are private acts of creation, even if encapsulated and hidden from one's conscious gaze. This is how the psyche makes a vivid contact, even if suffused with catastrophe and pain, with what it has lost. In the scene of "blank mourning," however, the psychic pain is not exiled into the body, but rather into action. Exile into action is a way of separating feeling from knowledge by erecting a wall between the mourner and his or her own pain. It is in front of this wall that Grossman's protagonist kneels in an attempt to release his dead son. He does not release him to life. He releases him in order to prevent his death from dying.

While fracture is associated with loss, healing entails the formation of language. In the Israeli domain of mourning the greatest challenge is exactly this: to constitute a language that releases the work of mourning from the prison of the collective language and its associated void; a language that confronts the terror of blank mourning with the endlessly specific hues of the private name, and the private grief.

Note

1 The Hebrew expression is: *Bemotam tsivu lanu et hahaim,* introduced by the poet H.N. Bialik, in 1898. Literally, it means: Dying, they bade us to live.

References

Amir, D. (2010). From mother tongue to language. *Psychoanalytic Review*, 97(4), 651–672.

Amir, D. (2014). *Cleft Tongue: The Language of Psychic Structures*. New-York and London: Karnac Books.

Amir, D. (2016a). When language meets the traumatic lacuna: The metaphoric, the metonymic and the psychotic modes of testimony. *Psychoanalytic Inquiry*, 36(8), 620–632.

Amir, D. (2016b). Hermetic narratives and false analysis: A unique variant of the mechanism of identification with the aggressor. *Psychoanalytic Review*, 103(4), 539–549.

Amir, D. (2018). *Bearing Witness to the Witness*: *A Psychoanalytic Perspective on Four Modes of Traumatic Testimony*. London & New-York: Routledge.

Amir, D. (2019). The bilingualism of the language of the victim and the language of the victimizer. *Psychoanalytic Dialogues*, 29(3), 367–381.

Amir, D. (2020). The bereaved survivor: Trauma survivors and blank mourning. *Psychoanalytic Perspectives*, 17(1), 74–83.

Bion, W.R. (1959). Attacks on linking. *International Journal of Psycho-Analysis*, 40, 308–315.

Bion, W.R. (1962a). *Learning from Experience*. New York: Basic Books.

Bion, W.R. (1962b). The psycho-analytic study of thinking. *International Journal of Psycho-Analysis*, 43, 306–310.

Bion, W.R. (1970). *Attention and Interpretation*. London: Tavistock.

Caruth, C. (1996). *Unclaimed Experience: Trauma Narrative and History*. Baltimore, MD: Johns Hopkins University Press.

Cohen-Fried, O. (2019). *And Who Will Remember Those Who Remember*. Tel-Aviv: Resling.

Derrida, J. (1995). *The Gift of Death* (trans: David Wills) Chicago, IL: The University of Chicago Press.

Durban, J. (2002). On love, hatred and anxiety–An introduction to Kleinian thinking. In *Melanie Klein–Selected Works*.

Freud, S. (1917). Mourning and Melancholia. *The Standard Edition of the Complete Psychological Works of Sigmund Freud, Volume XIV (1914–1916): On the History of the Psycho-Analytic Movement*. Papers on Metapsychology and Other Works, 237–258.

Gampel, Y. (1996). The interminable uncanny. In L. Rangell and R. Moses–Hrushovsky (eds.), *Psychoanalysis at the Political Border*. Madison: International Universities Press, pp. 85–98.

Gampel, Y. (2000). Reflections on the prevalence of the uncanny in social violence. In A. Robben and O. Surez-Orozco (eds.), *Cultures Under Siege: Collective Violence and Trauma in Interdiciplinary Perspectives*. Cambridge: Cambridge Univesity Press, pp. 48–69.

Gampel, Y. (2010). *Ces parentsq qui vivent à travers moi* (trans: T. Mishor) Jerusalem: Keter.

Garwood, A. (1996). The holocaust and the power of powerlessness: Survivor guilt an unhealed wound. *British Journal of Psychotherapy*, 13(2), 243–258.

Green, A. (1986). The analyst, symbolization, and absence in the analytic setting. In: *On Private Madness*. Madison, Conn. : International University Press.

Grossman, D. (2010). *Falling Out of Time*. Tel-Aviv: Hakibutz Hameuhad.

Jung, C.G. (1946). Psychology of the Transference. In *Collected Works*, 16 para 474.

Jung, C.G. (1952). Symbols of Transformation. In *Collected Works*, 5 para 89.

Kristeva, J. (1987). *Black Sun: Depression and Melancholia* (trans: Leon S. Roudiez). New-York: Columbia University Press.

Laub, D. (2005). Traumatic shutdown of narrative and symbolization. *Contemporary Psychoanalysis*, 41, 307–326.

Pontalis, J.–B. (1980). *Perdre de vue*. Paris: Gallimard.

Wardi, D. (1990). *Memorial Candles*. Jerusalem: Keter.

Chapter 4

The Experience of Voice in Analytic Listening

The infant's first cry on emerging from its mother's womb is also its first announcement of being there. This sound, in turn, evokes the mother's own vocal response: echoing the infant's cry, she wraps it in a vocal blanket which has a two-fold effect of soothing it as well as making it meaningful. But even before birth, the infant already communicates with what lies outside the womb through the sounds that reach it, whether originating from the mother's body or from the external world. The infant's first notion of the world is, in fact, a notion of sound: the mother's voice, her heartbeat, the sounds of people approaching her body and then turning away.

Anzieu in his book *The Skin Ego* (1989) discusses what he calls the "sound envelope" (p. 173), consisting alternately of the sounds produced by the environment and the sounds produced by the infant. The primary space is an acoustic one. Anzieu argues that prior to the visual dimension which Winnicott and Lacan emphasize in their work on the mirror stage and the mirror role of the mother, there is a "sound mirror" whose role is crucial for the new born's development. The new infant's most familiar sound is that of the scream, and Anzieu refers to four structurally and functionally distinct types of screams in a less than three weeks old infant: the scream of hunger, the scream of anger, the scream of pain (originating either inside or outside), and the scream of frustration. Each of these screams has its typical characteristics, but the scream of hunger is the most basic of the four, with the other three constituting variations of it. All these screams are pure physiological reflexes, triggering in the mother certain reactions which come to sooth them. Miraculously, the baby is most adequately calmed down by the mother's voice. From the second week of life, it is her voice that outdoes any other sound when it comes to pacifying the baby, outdoing even the visual presence of her face. From week three, another type

DOI: 10.4324/9781032715766-4

of scream emerges: the false distress scream, aiming to draw the mother's attention. This scream has a distinctly different physical structure than the preceding four ones. It is, in fact, the first intentional vocal communication, i.e., the first scream that is not a mere reflex. At five weeks, the infant picks out its mother's voice from among other voices, even though it is unable yet to visually distinguish her face. Between three and six months, the baby reaches the stage of babbling: it plays with the sounds it makes. Starting out with gurgles and crowing, the baby gradually trains its ability to differentiate, and willfully and stably produce the sounds that will come to make up its spoken language. Pre-lingual acquisition of meaning, which involves screaming and babbling, emerges before the acquisition of sub-lingual meaning–consisting of expressions and gestures. This is deeply connected to Anzieu's notion of the sound mirror. Even before the mother's gaze and smile reach it, the melodic bath (the mother's voice, her song, the music she plays) serves as a first sound mirror. The infant uses it initially by screaming (met, as said, by the mother's soothing voice), next by babbling, and eventually by means of articulation games (1985, pp. 175–178).

In her article "Sound Objects" (1995), Maiello writes that even before birth, the mother's voice, and the silences between the sounds it generates, furnish the fetus with a first prototype of the experience of presence and absence. Listening has a containing function resembling that of the skin as Bick (1968) described it: it is a precondition to the emergence of what Maiello calls the prenatal "sound object":

> The fetus receives and retains in its memory not only the melodious and rhythmical aspects of the mother tongue, but also the personal inflections and modulations of the maternal voice. If the child is capable, from inside its intrauterine sound-universe, of distinguishing the mother's voice from other sounds that reach it and is stimulated by its presence, we may hypothesize that some kind of a proto-dialogue begins at this early stage. [...] In other terms, the fetus' proto-mental nucleus [...], capable of transforming sensory information coming from external objects, could use the mother's voice for the creation of an internal object with sound qualities [...]. The absence of the voice on the other hand might give the child a proto experience of emptiness, of the emptied space in which thinking and language will develop and serve as instruments for re-evoking, i.e. 'giving voice again' to the lost object by naming it.
>
> (Maiello, 1995, p. 26)

Maiello later mentions that from the fourth month in utero, the fetus is able to stick its thumb into its mouth and suck it. This is an ability that appears when fetal hearing is fully developed. Would it be too farfetched to assume, she asks, that there is a link between the fetus' perception of the silence made by the absence of the mother's voice and the attempt to fill the gap by putting its thumb into its mouth? The disappearance of sound and the hollow of the mouth may merge into one and the same sensation. And while the fetus has no defense against the acoustic void by means of producing its own voice, it is quite able to fill the tactile void in the oral cavity. We may assume, Maiello argues, that the experience of the present and absent breast, which the schizoid-paranoid position splits into the good and the bad breast (Klein, 1946), has a prenatal antecedent associated with the present and absent maternal voice (Maiello, 1995, p. 27).

Maiello further adds that in addition to the present or absent maternal voice, the fetus is surrounded by a more general vocal ambience including the mother's body sounds and her heartbeat. This forms a continuous acoustic environment which is disrupted by birth. In this context she mentions how the presence and absence of a primary sound object, and the acoustic disruption of the continuous uterine ambience at the moment of birth, not only affect the newborn's ability to constitute good and continuous objects, but also make themselves known later in the therapeutic relationship. She thus points at the existence of a musical vertex of analytical attention, which takes account of the acoustic dimension of both the therapist's and the patient's presence:

> If it is true that a proto experience of rhythmical and musical consonance lies somewhere at the basis of every person's inner world, we can say that construction and reconstruction coincide in a unique event in the here and now of the session, so long as the transference relationship, whose means of communication is verbal language, is open both to the world of symbols and of sound.
>
> (Maiello, 1995, pp. 37–39)

I will use the above material as a point of departure, turning now to the constitution of the subject's vocal biography and its connection to the capacity for vocal reverie.

Vocal Biography, Vocal Reverie

Every person has a vocal biography which consists of one's ongoing experience of one's own voice as a continuity with whose fluctuations of volume he or she is familiar, as well as its specific nuances, its typical rhythm, pitch, and range of intensities.

Voice is affected by the speaker's physical and mental state at any given moment. It reflects, often even more than the bodily experience, signs of tiredness, fear, or distress. Yet despite momentary collapses, voice constitutes a flow, a continuity. The vocal biography is a kind of vocal map which represents what is fixed and what changes, serving as a type of vocal mirror for the one who speaks. Much like the mother learns to differentiate between the child's screams, as Anzieu has put it, the subject himself, too, comes to distinguish between the various registers of his or her own voice and identify their meanings. One learns to tell the difference between a certain vibration in the vocal cords which announces excitement, and another slightly different vibration which indicates fear. One learns to tell apart the rhythms and changing pitch of speech: high and restless when trying to avoid listeners' picking up certain gaps and lacunae in one's knowledge, for instance, while resonant and stable when dwelling securely in the idea one conveys. Truth and falsehood have different vocal registers. This becomes more complicated of course when truth or falsehood are not intentional and conscious, and what we are dealing with are links and attacks on linking (Bion, 1959) which largely escape the speaker's own awareness.

When I turned eight my father, an experienced music teacher, gave me an ancient Japanese poem as a birthday present:

> The deer on pine mountain,
> Where there are no falling leaves,
> Knows the coming of autumn
> Only by the sound of his own voice.
>
> Nakatomi No Yoshinobu (10th century)

It was his way to tell me how he listened: music, for him, was not a score consisting of sounds imparted from the outside in. It was more like a score which, in parallel to its external orchestration, was also orchestrated and performed within. More than that: he studied the musical qualities by what they resonated inside him. What he taught me through this poem had to do not only with listening to music, but also with listening to any score as such. This might be called the witnessing function (Amir, 2012) of the voice: when there is no objective, external signs, the deer–and much like him, the human psyche–will testify to events on the basis of the echo chamber of their own voice. The witnessing function of the voice is the way in which the voice itself serves as a "third", creating for the person producing it a kind of "vantage point" that testifies to his emotional state. Thus, a two-way relationship is formed between the voice and the speaker: not only the person speaks through the voice–but the very voice returns an echo which serves, for the speaker, as a witness.

Ogden (1995), in a chapter focusing on forms of vitality and death in the transference and countertransference, writes about a patient whom he experienced as indifferent or emotionally blocked for a long time:

> I could hear the voice with which I was speaking to myself at that moment in the meeting as the voice of a person experiencing a sense of impenetrable alienation from Mrs. S; at the same time, I also recognized something else in that voice for the first time. It was the voice of a spurned lover.
>
> (Ibid., p. 707)

Once he recognizes the spurned lover in his own voice, he has an insight into both the patient's feelings of love for him, and his own love for the patient. This part of the musical score of their relations, however, was not explicit. It was communicated precisely and only in this way. Here Ogden deploys what we may call a "vocal reverie": a form of attention to a voice not merely as internal but also as one that echoes the external.

Voice is one of the primary enigmas. Much before the language which the mother uses to turn to her baby, her voice stimulates the infant to become familiar with its nuances and movements, and the infant is driven to translate it–in Laplanche's (1989[1987], p. 20) terms–into a meaningful score. Throughout life, and in any human encounter, the voice continues to present an enigma asking for translation. The next sections will discuss two different pathological positionings on the vocal spectrum, attempting to cast light on the complex nature of the work of its translation in the therapeutic space.

Adhesive Vocal Identification in Autistic States

Meltzer's (1975a, 1975b) concept of "adhesive identification" refers to autistic children's difficulty in attaining a three-dimensional experience of the object which is required for creating the function of containing. In order to feel that the object is a container which has a capacity to hold, we must experience it as three-dimensional. At the same time, in order to internalize it, we must also perceive ourselves as three dimensional. Within two-dimensional relations the object is experienced as inseparable from its sensory features. This is why autistic children actually cling to their objects. They touch the people around them continuously and inappropriately since in their experience people exist or are present only through contact with their external surfaces. Adhesive identification, namely the defensive cling-ing to the object, serves to lessen the anxiety of breakdown. Autistic chil-dren do not experience themselves as three-dimensional just as they don't experience others as such. Their self, too, is experienced only in terms of its external features and not as having an interior. The defensive adhesion to the other is an attempt to alleviate the anxiety of disintegration through the artificial adoption of the other's facial expressions, body movements, or vocal gestures, i.e., to use this other person's external surface as though they were one's own. This is an actual adhesion of bits of the other's surface to the person's own deficient surface, enacting in that way the wish to stick parts of the other's identity onto one's perforated self. This ongoing friction with the other has a twofold purpose: it comes to keep the other present, since as soon as there is no friction, the other feels absent, and it also aims to keep the self present by means of the sense of outline this friction sup-plies. Judith Mitrani, in her paper "On Adhesive Pseudo-Object Relations" (1994), elaborates on the notion of an archaic mode of object-relating, in which "adhesive equation" rather than true identification predominates; in which the superimposition of subject and object is so complete, continuous and chronic that the concepts of "otherness" and of "space" have little or no relevance. Instead, the awareness of space and otherness present the subject with an unbearable experience of utter catastrophe and a threat to a sense of "going-on-being".

The term "adhesive vocal identification", which I suggest here, refers to a situation when one person sticks a "voice patch" belonging to another person onto the damaged surface of his or her own voice. When the vocal continuum is experienced as perforated, lacking any sense of an ongoing vocal biography–the need arises to cover the voice's torn and cracked parts with pieces of the other's voice. This does not refer to the more common ways in which one voice is affected by another–for instance, the fact that when we speak with someone who has a foreign accent, that accent sometimes seems to get itself briefly stuck onto our own speech, or the fact that when we are in conversation with someone who is speaking in a particularly low voice we tend to naturally lower our own voice in return. Nor am I speaking of the phenomenon of incorporation of the other's voice (for instance, when in certain situations we find ourselves reproducing our parents' voice, a kind of enacted recollection), or the internalization of the other's voice (which we carry inside while it is saturated with the hues of our personal vocal biography). A vocal adhesive identification is the attaching of one voice to another with extremely coarse stitches. This is a primitive imitation, a kind of "imitation without an imitator" following Bion's (1970, p. 102) "thought without a thinker" which he considers typical of primitive non-thinking. It includes every singular parameter of the other's voice: its pitch, volume, pace–but without the sense or presence of a voice's owner. And since it is the role of the voice owner, in natural speech, to maintain the natural relations between these vocal parameters–an arbitrary relationship will emerge between them when he or she is absent. The result will be a coarse adhesion of the other's voice to that of the speaker, in which the other's voice is present as a foreign body: it can neither be swallowed nor ejected because there is no interior that can digest or refuse it.

In Anzieu's (1989) and Maiello's (1995) terms, the autistic structure can be considered as a primitive, organic lack in the vocal envelope, leading to an acoustic void which vocal adhesive identification seeks to fill. As the autistic infant experiences neither itself nor the other as three-dimensional, there is neither an experience of the self as an acoustic container which can absorb the maternal voice, nor an experience of a maternal acoustic container taking in the infant's voice. The only way to create an illusion of a sound envelope or of a sound mirror is the adhesive clinging to the other's voice.

Another typical autistic way of filling the acoustic void is the phenomenon of echolalia, which may be thought of as another form of adhesion. Echolalia is a type of echoing: the autistic person's repeating what the other says, but in a manner that is neither communicative nor appropriate. For instance, in response to the question "Do you want to drink something?"—the autistic person, rather than producing an answer, will repeat the question. This is an immediate echolalia. In delayed echolalia, the autistic person may ask: "Do you want to drink something?" sometime later, when he or she feels thirsty.

For autistic children, language is a form of auto-sensuousness. They can lean or rub themselves against words, but they cannot use them to communicate. This is why autistic children prefer consonants, which are felt more clearly in the mouth. Similarly, they will be attracted by rigid forms of rhyme, due to the identical, repeated and invariable sounds it makes in the mouth, offering them a rigid "surface" against which they can lean (Amir, 2013). The adhesive vocal identification involves all of these: the patches of the other person's voice do not carry specific meaning or any distinctive content. They have musical and tactile qualities, instead, and they are chosen for the degree of sensory gratification they can supply and the way they suit the purpose of the immediate filling of the acoustic void.

An important distinction, here, must be made between "false voice" and adhesive vocal identification. False voice refers to the adopting of vocal features that fit in with the other's or the surroundings' expectations or needs, and therefore constitutes a type of camouflage of an inner conflict between what the subject experiences and what she or he perceives as desirable. The resulting voice is rather mechanical: it resembles the sound of the electric keyboard compared to a grand piano. Since it does not originate in the speaker's sound-box, its affect remains flat and incapable of evoking an emotional response in the other. Adhesive vocal identification, however, does not camouflage an existing state of affairs but rather aims to circumscribe a void. The sound this adhesion produces, therefore, is not just merely flat in terms of its resonance: it rather subverts the very essence of sound as such. Not only is it shorn of any of the speaker's specific musical characteristics (like the false voice in which pitch, rhythm and volume entertain artificial relations): it lacks any musical features whatsoever. Under adhesive vocal identification, the parameters of voice stayed rigid in their original state and got transplanted, as such, without any transformation or context, to the speaker's voice. This resembles what happens when the autistic child, when asked "Are you hungry?", will reply: "Are you hungry?"—without any syntactic transformation of person—from "you" to "I"—or of intonation—from question to assertion. The adhesion of the other's voice to that of the speaker takes place without any process of digestion or internalization of that voice. It is rather stuck on, just as it is, with pitch, volume and pace of the spoken segment remaining unchanged.

Case Illustration[1]

When Naomi, an autistic young woman, begins psychotherapy, what strikes me most is her bizarre response to my words. She relates to them in a sensual way–rather than verbally or symbolically. She rubs against them, tastes, and chews them, but never "thinks" of them. This turns our entire discourse into an uncanny one, like a walk through an unknown terrain in which the usual rules of reality or even those of inner reality do not obtain. She does not anticipate what I am saying as a listener, but rather like an animal waiting to pounce on her prey: she closely follows the motions of my lips, the sound of my words; she sniffs the intervals between them, "swallows" or "laps up" what I say in the most concrete sense of these terms as though they are foods, sweets, a bitter pill. She never adds anything of her own. Instead, she repeats what I say with my exact intonation. Her eagerness to hear my words does not seem related to what they mean but rather to the very contact they enable her with me. It seems connected with the simple physical fact that I am talking to her, that my lingual surface is there, stable enough to let her rest her own lingual surface against it. She is not trying to "swallow" my words as a primitive form of incorporation. Rather, she treats the words themselves, especially the consonants and the vowels within every word, as inanimate objects which she scratches against her tongue, chews, or spits out.

Alvarez (1992) writes about the moment in which she understood that Robbi, an autistic patient, was experiencing one stimulus in terms of another: a voice (an auditory stimulus) in terms of a colour (a visual stimulus). Naomi experiences my voice in terms of taste. There are "tasty words" against "bitter words that you must swallow". No logical link can be identified between what she experiences as tasty and the word's objective content. These idiosyncratic bizarre differentiations are connected more than anything else to the relation between consonants and vowels within every word: a multi-consonant word is experienced as tasty, while a word that has more vowels is experienced as "bitter" or "disgusting". Multi-consonant words that rhyme are the tastiest.

Naomi treats me as a fluffy surface that could be ignored or passed through. If I "give her tasty words" she gazes at me for a moment, hoping for more. Otherwise, she detaches herself, or gazes through me. More and more often I feel that what seems like a speech which is directed at me–or a game that she is playing with me–is an autistic act that is aimed to block any recognition of my separateness (and the acoustic void related to it), as well as any possibility of creating living relationships with me.

Naomi is the eldest daughter of three. During her mother's pregnancy she suffered a severe stress which finally caused a premature delivery, one month before the anticipated date. Naomi was born with the umbilical cord wrapped around her neck, barely breathing, and remained hospitalized for two months after her birth. The mother suffered from a post-natal psychotic depression, refused to see Naomi or hold her and was convinced that the baby was "Satan" who was born to destroy her. Following an intensive psychiatric treatment, the mother began to recover and started taking care of the baby but was not allowed to be alone with her until Naomi was one year old. The father, a hard worker, was usually absent for most of the day and was not available for either his daughter or his wife. The only person who steadily took care of Naomi during her first year was the maternal grandmother, to whom she was deeply attached. When Naomi was about one year and a half the grandmother had a severe stroke (during which she fainted in front of her little granddaughter), after which she was hospitalized in a rehabilitation institute and never regained the ability to speak. Following the event, Naomi's mother went through another period of major depression. At the time of the grandmother's stroke Naomi already spoke a few words and was physically developed and active. A few months after the event her parents noticed that she became introverted and withdrawn, that her language did not develop properly for her age and that the few sentences that she did say sounded bizarre both in shape and in content. She was ascribed to a special school for children with communication difficulties. At school, too, she was quite withdrawn. Her mother, who gave birth to twins (a boy and a girl) when Naomi was four years old, felt relieved when Naomi shut herself in her room and preferred that she would not demand her attention. Whenever she did try to play with her–Naomi used to cling to the mother's body in a very disturbing manner, arousing in her both fear and disgust.

On her 12th birthday Naomi lay down on a train track, waiting quietly for the train to come and simply "take her away from there". She could not say (not then, not in retrospect) anything about this except that this "there" was not pain, or loneliness or anything else with a name, a form, or content. "There" was the region which was not "here". She was then referred to a behavioral psychotherapist and stayed with him for almost eight years. The treatment ended when he moved to another town, and she was then referred to me.

The idiom "there" repeated itself through many years of treatment. I noticed that in many instances Naomi says "I am there" while she intends to say "I am here" (for example, whenever she enters my office). In many instances she asks me to "come and sit there" while, in fact, she wants me to come and sit close to her. Interestingly, Alvarez describes a moment of progress in Robbi's treatment when he was finally able to make a wish to be "there", namely when he could imagine a place that was not here and now (Alvarez, 1992, p. 63). In an opposite manner, what I felt with Naomi was that there is no "here" that is available for her. While Robbi could not hold in mind the possibility of another place–and could only relate to the concrete and the actual–Naomi could not have any vivid experience of the "here and now". She was "there", detached from any "living company" (Alvarez, 1992) or common experience. "There" is a zone of neither life nor death, neither past nor future, hence not a living present either. "There" is what will never be "here".

For a long period of time, I felt as though I was walking through a swamp, a dense, sticky space in which words stretched sideways, became kneadable, bounced or were thrown back and forth–but never created discourse. At times I felt as an object myself, which Naomi, unbeknownst to herself, was throwing back and forth. Between sessions she used to send me repetitive, meaningless text messages, as if she was using me to fill up the hole which I created by being absent. All this was accompanied by a strange sense that whatever was happening between us was not happening "here", that is, in a breathing, vivid present.

How do we turn "there" into "here"? How do we turn the adhesive vocal identification into a polyphony? Suzanne Maiello quotes Novalis who writes beautifully: "Disease is a musical problem. Cure is a musical solution" (Novalis[2] in Maiello, 1995). If the adhesive vocal identification is the musical problem–what is the musical solution?

As a result of a mixture of organic and environmental reasons, Naomi reacted in an autistic encapsulation to a situation in which–besides an extremely traumatic birth–she experienced a violent separation both from her grandmother, to whom, as said, she was deeply attached, and from her mother with whom her initial bonding was extremely fragile. Her clinging to the sensual aspects of words instead of creating them as agents of meaning–was related to the fact that the "sound-envelope" she generated that way protected her from fragmentation and from being violently penetrated both by the outside as well as by her own internal world.

The autistic dyad she formed with me was one in which we stayed "side by side" without being connected–and therefore without acknowledging our separateness. In a certain sense, her unconscious intention was to create a scene in which I was "glued" to her (through her repeating of the sounds I made) without acknowledging me as a separate subject. Her clinging to me (much as her clinging to her mother's body) was an effort to adhere to my surface without enabling a link between our interiors. The therapeutic mission, therefore, was to enable the connection between our inner worlds–hoping that the inner connection would gradually soften her need to glue our surfaces. This began with my refusal to cooperate with her endless uninterrupted sound chains, which strengthened the illusion of a common surface, and continued with my insistence to bring myself into the session in a manner that would not allow the continuous gluing of our surfaces as a substitute to relationships. In musical terms it can be said that I insisted on creating, despite Naomi's vocal adhesive identification and vocal clinging– a polyphony of my own–inviting Naomi to also create one herself.

One of the most touching illustrations of this process was when one day she brought in a looper: a special recording machine which created an echo of what was just recorded. For example, having recorded "how are you?", the machine would create an endless loop of "how are you? How are you? How are you?" until we recorded something else–which also repeated itself endlessly until we interrupted it with a new one. Naomi was extremely fascinated by this instrument and was willing to listen to the loops of her voice for the whole session. The endless repetition calmed and rocked her, and she listened to it with her eyes closed. At a certain moment I suggested a game in which I stopped abruptly the loop by recording a new sound of my own, inviting her to do the same, to surprise me, to change. Naomi protested at first and was furious with the unexpected interruption, but very slowly, she was carried away. What was recorded eventually was an orchestra of both our voices: high pitched, low pitched, asking and laughing. This beautiful musical texture, which Naomi called "the choir of us"–was a first sign of the possibility to create psychic music in a place that had been under the sway of anti-musical rules.

Here, as often in cases of adhesive vocal identification, the mutative interpretation was not an interpretation, not even a primitive one, "*of* the voice" (by this I mean any verbal interpretation of vocal behaviors, like "You are sticking your voice unto mine so there will be no gap between us; a gap is scary"). Such an interpretation could be appropriate at a later stage. But to get to that stage, an interpretative "step" first needed to be created, one that takes the shape of what I call "voice-based interpretation" or "interpretation *through* the voice". This type of interpretation is as close as possible to the actual craft of gluing and separating. Rather than commenting "about adhesion" or "about the fear of void"–one slowly puts apart the stuck-together regions by creating a breathing acoustic space. The first stage in the creation of this acoustic space is the creation of a living acoustic envelope (by means of the therapist's acoustic presence). The second stage is the creation of an acoustic mirror (through the echoing of the patient's sounds). Only in the final stage an acoustic dialogue comes into existence, one between two vocal subjects.

Stern (2010, p. 139), referring to music therapy as described by Tony Wigram (2004), marks the following therapeutic elements or stages:

1. Mirroring, imitation and copying: the therapist uses his instrument to reproduce exactly what the patient just played–its vitality form, rhythm, melody, etc.
2. Matching: Selective and partial imitation. The dynamic features of the music the patient just produced are maintained, but other features are altered. This is essentially a musically based affect attunement, which resembles the affect attunement between parent and child.
3. Empathic improvisation: the therapist improvises a response that reflects (without imitation or attunement) the emotional state of the patient.
4. Grounding, holding, and containing: the therapist creates a stable musical anchor–a steady pulsed beat, for instance, which provides a dynamic framework within which the patient's improvisation can work.
5. Dialoguing: turn taking back-and-forth without unduly long breaks[3] and without interruptions by the two participants.

6. Accompanying: the therapist provides an accompaniment that is different from what the patient is playing but lies "dynamically underneath the patient's music" (Wigram, 2004, p. 106).

Unsurprisingly, work with vocal adhesive identification uses a considerable part of these elements. This is because we are dealing with early communicational pathologies preceding symbolic language. Communication, when using these elements, can be conducted mainly via the voice, and the therapeutic work with the voice employs it in a manner very much like the music therapist uses musical instruments. In the latter case, however, there are usually two subjects who play their instruments, whereas in the therapeutic work with vocal adhesive identification we are dealing with a patient who is a pre-subject rather than subject, and who, lacking a voice or any ability to play, uses the other's voice as a replacement of his or her own "vocal instrument". In this situation, the therapeutic work must create the basic conditions for the patient to experience her or his voice as their own instrument, long before they are able to play with it in the shared acoustic space. Only in this way the vocal adhesive identification will turn from what blocks communication and thinking to what enables the experience of *being here* and *being within*.

The Psychotic Split Between Voice and Meaning

Aulagnier (2001) addresses in her writings, as mentioned earlier, several factors that may foretell psychotic potentiality. The first is the absence of the father from the discourse of the "word-bearer" (the mother), an absence that leaves the infant exposed to the incestuous contents that the mother was unable to repress and from which the very presence of the father did not shield it. The second factor is the mother's failure to repress her incestuous wish directed at her own mother (expressed, see Chapter 2, in her unconscious wish to give her own child to her mother, thus repeat her own birth through him rather than let him be a subject in his own right). The third factor is related to the identificatory void caused by the mother's inability to provide historical and emotional context for the preverbal experiences inscribed in the infant's body, experiences which the infant is unable to remember. The fourth factor is the mother's refusal to allow the infant its separate existence and its own thoughts. Her need to understand and to articulate every psychic zone denies the infant's right to privacy and autonomous thinking, turning it into a sort of satellite-object utterly subjected to her authority. The mechanism of repression which is typical of neurotic development is replaced here by the mechanism of denial which is typical of psychotic development. While the mother has not repressed that which must be repressed (her wish for the death or un-birth of her child)–what has not been repressed must not be exposed to either the infant or herself. The fear of breaching the prohibition imposed upon knowing invokes a sense of catastrophe in the child whenever it draws close to an understanding. The prohibition to understand may turn into a prohibition to assimilate any experience into memory, thus creating "holes in memory" where entire parts of the subject's history are erased.

When there is no maternal voice telling the subject its historical narrative, the infant confronts an intolerable void. It then fills this void with a primitive delusional structure, which comes to replace the proper causal order of the common discourse and the common rules of speech and thinking. The child, in other words, copes with the void stemming from the absence of an ongoing experience of self, by creating a delusional structure. This could be seen as a means of restoring a previously prohibited autonomy, at the price of its turning into an underground one, far away both from the mother's and the public's eyes. In this sense, the psychotic's delusion may be seen as an expression of his or her struggle for the right to exist (Aulagnier, 2001). The defense of the psychotic child occurs by way of an attack on both the presence of voice and the presence of meaning, and even more so by an attack on the unity of voice and meaning–a monstrous union representing the link to primary unrepressed prohibitions. Such an attack creates blind spots related to contents that have not been repressed by the mother–and that the infant is not permitted to see, to think or to remember[4] (Amir, 2010). Thus, the psychotic acoustic void is different than its autistic version. While the latter is the outcome of organic failure in the internalization of the vocal envelope and in the use of the maternal vocal mirror, the former involves a primary rupture between the mother's voice, which communicates the truth of her non-wish for a child, and her words whose message contradicts what the voice conveys. This rupture makes it impossible for the child to either experience the primary dyad as a meaningful acoustic space or internalize a fluent vocal biography, either of the mother or of itself. The solution is the development of a delusional acoustic space, which on the one hand prevents the experience of the acoustic void, and on the other hand prevents the encounter with the intolerable truth. We can, in this sense, consider the psychotic split between voice and meaning as, simultaneously, an internalization of the mother's psychotic split (as said, she dissociates the emotional message from the words into which she pours it)–and a defense against the encounter with this split.

In a chapter discussing failures in the acoustic envelope, Anzieu (1989) writes that one can often identify the mother of the schizophrenic patient by the features of her voice: it tends to be monotonous (lacking in tempi), metallic (lacking in melody), confusing and invasive. This results in a perforated "sound-bath" (ibid., p. 224). Where the acoustic mirror which the mother offers her child is pathogenic, it displays, according to Anzieu, the following types of defect: it is out of tune–in the sense of behaving in contradiction with what the baby feels, expects, or expresses; it is sudden–shifting between one extreme and the other in a way that is arbitrary and remains unintelligible to the baby, causing repeated micro-traumas to its emerging stimulus barrier; and finally, it is indifferent and remote.

Following Anzieu we may, therefore, think of the defensive split that the psychotic person creates between voice and meaning as his or her way of disconnecting the pathogenic, delusive maternal sound mirror, turning it into a "sound wall," a detached, foreign sound object that is neither associated with the infant's figure nor reflects the infant's image.

Case Illustration[5]

Benjamin, in his early twenties, was referred to therapy by his psychiatrist. He is a handsome young man, but his facial expression is sealed, and his gestures are bizarre. He inserts fingers into his mouth as he speaks seemingly trying to push the words back in, instead of uttering them out loud. The few sentences he utters usually end with the words "I don't know." This is not a coincidental combination of words. Benjamin refuses to know and no less refuses to become attached. He is not formally diagnosed as schizophrenic, but his interpersonal discourse does not follow normative emotional and linguistic rules. He usually speaks in broken sentences, mumbling, as if speaking to himself rather than to his interlocutor, looking at the ceiling or floor, and rolling his eyes. It appears that his understanding of the other's discourse, too, doesn't correspond with the latter's intentions; what he hears is usually different from what was said, mostly with a paranoid shade indicating a faulty reality testing. His tone of voice is dull and monotonous, showing no affect, lacking any signs of punctuation.

His appearance is as strange as his speech. He wears short-sleeved shirts even on the coldest of winter days, mostly inside-out. When I ask about that he replies, as usual, that he doesn't know why, but that's how it has always been. I understand that wearing a shirt inside-out is similar to his pushing words in rather than out, or to the way he constructs a non-language rather than one that makes sense. He is extremely unkempt and dirty, neglects his body and doesn't treat any physical problem, not even when he is in pain. One day, arriving with his face swollen, he tells me that his teeth ache. When I ask him why he doesn't have them treated he replies that he can't stand for anyone to push fingers into his mouth. I suddenly realize that psychotherapy, too, is a way of shoving fingers into his mouth, into his cavities of speech or deeper yet, wondering whether the reason he speaks with his fingers deep in his mouth is also connected to his unwillingness to allow me to insert my own fingers (or words) there.

Benjamin describes his mother as a hard, persecutory, and intrusive woman who had not only despised him since his early years for his strangeness and peculiarity but also never listened to his signs of distress. His father is perceived as weak, dependent, almost voiceless regarding the mother's high, shrill voice–which Benjamin claims he cannot bear. Speaking to her on the telephone, he feels like flinging the phone down to escape the awful vibrations that her voice conveys to him. Often, he can't even recall what she said to him, being so preoccupied with the attempt not to hear her voice. When I ask what is so troubling about her voice he mumbles: "It's like inserting a bug into your ear. It hurts your ear. You can't bear it. You simply can't."

Aulagnier (2001) claims in a similar context that the fact that hearing cannot seal itself off (the child cannot "shut" its ears) accentuates the persecutory character of the voice typical of psychosis. The psychotic has no escape from the tormenting voice, neither by understanding the uttered content (since understanding is prohibited) nor by hushing the voice itself.

One day, Benjamin arrived at our appointment a few minutes early, and while standing in the lane by my house my dog barked at him. Being in the garden, behind a fence, it posed no danger to Benjamin. Nevertheless, when he entered my office, he was more upset than I'd ever seen him before, stuttering that he hated dogs, mumbling broken sentences, fingers deep in his mouth, about a student who once set fire to his neighbor's dog because its barking had disturbed his studies for a mid-term exams.

I understood that he was telling me something about the intensity of his hatred and rage, about his jealousy of anyone I love, perhaps even warning me against his homicidal wish towards whoever takes his place or threatens it. At the same time, I sensed he was also telling me something about the meaning of noise for him. The dog's barking, piercing his ears without his being able to defend against it, provoked the same helpless rage that his mother's voice used to provoke. His homicidal wish towards it was his homicidal wish towards his mother as well as towards me for not stopping the barking and preventing the voice's intrusiveness. The intrusion of voice preceded the intrusion of meaning and was much more difficult for him. He used to disassemble meaning by fragmenting sentences, by his erasing of my questions each time anew with the "I don't know" by which he ended every utterance. The voice, however, was much more difficult to nullify. It penetrated under his skin. Long before he could understand what his mother was saying to him, her voice was an insupportable, unbearable stimulus. It was that unbearable stimulus against which he set up a psychotic barrier, the only defense he could afford against that intrusion. The psychotic language produced a haven in which, while not sheltered from her voice, he was beyond the reach of her insights. His finger-shoving into his mouth indicated that the gesture of disarming the voice was also displaced to his own voice and words and was also enacted within the therapeutic relations with me. Not only was it hard to hear his voice, but it was also extremely difficult to understand the words he uttered. In other words, since he couldn't shut *his* ears against *my* voice, he shut *my* ears against *his* voice.

The type of interpretive approach I used with Benjamin, was one I would call "interpretation *of* the voice". The only interpretations to which Benjamin was able to respond were the ones which were experience-near and adjusted to his primary developmental stage: "You are pushing your voice inside so it won't come out," or "When I am talking too much you feel me getting right into your ear, and you need to stop me so your ear will stop hurting," or again: "You're speaking in a quiet voice so I won't hear you and understand what it is you're saying." These interpretations came, first, to point at the split off voice as such ("You are pushing your voice inside, so it won't come out"). Only then, gradually, they began to offer the very beginning of meaning ("You're speaking in a quiet voice, so

I won't hear you and understand what it is you're saying"). Benjamin never responded verbally to these interpretations. Rather, his response revealed itself through the changes in his vocal parameters. As time went by, his monotonous voice transformed into a more dynamic graph of volume, timbre, and pace. These were first, cautious signs of his increasing ability to use my voice as a sound mirror and to play in the acoustic space our relationship supplied. More and more, as time passed, these signs revealed the fact that behind his vocal blockage, or "sound wall," a living voice was still hiding, looking for a way to make itself heard.

Conclusion

At the end of a case presentation in Amsterdam, 20 years ago, a young Italian psychoanalyst commented: "I have tears in my ears." Besides speaking in a foreign language, maybe confusing between eyes and ears, he might also have precisely meant this: it was his ears, rather than his eyes, that filled up with tears.

While our eyes are often filled up with tears in response to content—one may say that our ears are filled up with tears in response to sound. The response to sound is similar to the response to smell. It is immediate, it precedes contact with the content of the spoken words, it does not pass through any rational or intellectual processing. Sound, like smell, has the power to immediately throw us in, or backward, to evoke memories and revive forgetfulness. The importance of using the acoustic dimension of the analytic space is therefore related to the fact that within this space the analytic duo has access not only to the deepest internal dramas–but also to the most natural ways of repair.

Notes

1 This case illustration is partly based on its previous publication in: Amir, D. (2013). The psychic organ point of autistic syntax. *Journal of Child Psychotherapy, 39*(1), 3–21.
2 https://quotefancy.com/quote/1346880/Novalis-Every-disease-is-a-musical-problem-Its-cure-a-musical-solution-The-more-rapid-and
3 Perhaps to avoid what I mentioned earlier as "acoustic void".
4 My intention is not to claim that the mother is the cause of the child's psychosis, but rather to suggest that for reasons related both to the actual maternal presence and to the way the child constructs her presence–the internalized mother acts in

a way that the child experiences as attacking both his freedom and his ability to think.

5 This case illustration is partly based on the following paper:

Amir, D. (2010). The split between voice and meaning: The dual function of psychotic syntax. *International Forum of Psychoanalysis, 19*(1), 34–42.

References

Alvarez, A. (1992). *Live Company: Psychotherapy with Autistic, Borderline, Deprived and Abused Children*. London: Routledge.

Amir, D. (2010). The split between voice and meaning: The dual function of psychotic syntax. *International Forum of Psychoanalysis*, 19(1), 34–42.

Amir, D. (2012). The inner witness. *International Journal of Psycho-analysis*, 93, 879–896.

Amir, D. (2013). The psychic organ point of autistic syntax. *Journal of Child Psychotherapy*, 39(1), 3–21.

Anzieu, D. (1989). *The Skin Ego*. New Haven: Yale University Press.

Aulagnier, P. (2001). *The Violence of Interpretation* (trans: Alan Sheridan). London: Routledge.

Bick, E. (1968). The experience of the skin in early object-relations. *International Journal of Psycho-Analysis*, 49, 484–486.

Bion, W. (1959). Attacks on linking. *International Journal of Psycho-Analysis*, 40, 308–315.

Bion, W. (1970). *Attention and interpretation*. London: Tavistock.

Klein, M. (1946). Notes on some schizoid mechanisms. *The International Journal of Psychoanalysis*, 27, 99–110.

Laplanche, J. (1989[1987]). *New Foundations for Psychoanalysis* (trans: D. Macey). Oxford: Blackwell.

Maiello, S. (1995). The sound-object: A hypothesis about prenatal auditory experience and memory. *Journal of Child Psychotherapy*, 21, 23–41.

Meltzer, D. (1975a). Dimensionality as a parameter of mental functioning: its relation to narcissistic organization. In D. Meltzer, J. Bremner, S. Hoxter, D. Weddell, and I. Wittenberg (eds.), *Explorations in Autism*. Strath Tay: Clunie Press, pp. 223–238.

Meltzer, Donald. (1975b). Adhesive identification. *Contemporary Psycho-Analysis*, 11, 289–310.

Mitrani, J.L. (1994). On adhesive pseudo-object relations. *Contemporary Psychoanalysis*, 30(2), 348–366.

Ogden, T.H. (1995). Analysing forms of aliveness and deadness of the transference-countertransference. *International Journal of Psychoanalysis*, 76, 695–709.

Stern, D. (2010). *Forms of Vitality: Exploring Dynamic Experience in Psychology, the Arts, Psychotherapy, and Development*. Oxford: Oxford University Press.

Wigram, T. (2004). *Improvisation: Methods and Techniques for Music Therapy Clinicians, Educators and Students*. London: Jessica Kingsley Publishers.

Chapter 5

From "Turning-Away" to "Turning-To"

Adoption as Radical Hospitality

My deep connection with the subject of adoption is related to my being the mother of a son born in St Petersburg, Russia, whom I adopted when he was nearly one year old. This chapter combines theoretical thoughts and clinical materials with passages of personal memoir. It might be considered an attempt to manage the big cracks presenting themselves on the adoption of a child, and to face them employing both "metonymical witnessing", located in the first person and in the *experiencing I*, and "metaphorical witnessing", which creates a constant movement between the first person and the third person, or between the *experiencing I* and the *reflective I* (Amir, 2016, 2019).

In her book *The Adoption Life Cycle* (1992) Elinor Rosenberg writes that one of the great illusions concerning adoption is that it offers the fantasy of the perfect solution, both for the biological parents, who feel unable to raise the child they just had, and the adoptive parents who want to raise a child but cannot have one, as well as for the child himself, who is in desperate need of a home. This ostensibly perfect solution, however, is what none of the parties ever wanted (ibid). Biological parents would have preferred to be able to bring up their own child; most adoptive parents would rather raise their own biological children, and adopted children would have preferred for the parents who raise them to be the same parents who gave birth to them.

Elsewhere she writes about how even when the process has evolved in the best possible way–and both the parents and the child are happy–there will always be present, between them, the knowledge that somewhere out there the biological parents are mourning the child they could not raise themselves, a knowledge that haunts the alleged sense of perfection (ibid.). In adoption, therefore, unlike in the case of giving birth, deep processes of mourning are always included: those of the parents, those of the child, and

DOI: 10.4324/9781032715766-5

those of the unspoken ghosts, long before the bonding that must contain such processes of mourning has even had a chance to develop.

Various authors have called the inner representation of the birth parent in the context of adopted children a "hole object" (Quinodoz, 1996, p. 324), "lost object" (Deeg, 1989, p. 152), or "phantom object" (Rosenberg & Horner, 1991, p. 73).

What is the difference between mourning a real object and mourning a phantom object? Rachel Sopher (2018) suggests the notion of a mental "phantom pain" associated with the removal of a mental organ. To allow the self to survive a premature experience of separation, a mental part under-goes "amputation" and becomes disconnected from the other parts of the psyche so that contact with it is lost. The only remaining sign of its exist-ence is in the form of "phantom pains": pains whose source is unknown or unthinkable and which are not amenable to treatment (ibid.).

But a phantom *object* is not just the result of amputation from the psy-chic body: it is an object that never attained the status of a real, mourn-able object. The hole such an object causes in the fabric of the infantile mind lacks outline in many ways and is therefore immeasurable. Thus, even though the difference between babies who have been adopted immediately after birth and babies who spent months and sometimes years in institutions before being adopted is huge–they do share the experience of a phantom object of the biological parent.

Not only the adopted children's work of mourning but also the adoptive parents' work of mourning links back to a phantom object. Adoptive par-ents, too, find themselves coping with an infantile phantom object that lacks concrete boundaries: first–except for in the case of "ideological adoption", when the family decided to adopt a child for social, moral reasons–every adopted child is, to an extent, a substitute for a biological child who wasn't born, a "phantom child" who functions as an ideal prototype. And while all parenting can be associated with concessions in view of held prototypes of both ideal parent and ideal child–the concessions involved in adoption are far greater. Therefore, the adopted child's work of mourning parallels, at least up to a point, that of the adoptive parent: in both cases it concerns a phantasmatic object whose abstract nature causes it to grow infinite, lacking concrete, realistic outlines; and so in both cases mourning is not about a real object but rather about an idea of unconditional closeness, of natural, effort-less love that does not need to strain to cover genetic and biographical gaps.

In addition, the adoptive parents are forced to deal with the phantom object of the biological parents. Quite a few of the adoptive parents I have met over the years were preoccupied, no less than the children themselves, with the identities of their adoptive children's biological parents. They shifted between arrogant contempt, blaming these parents not only for the difficulties their adopted children experienced but also for their presumable genetic imperfections, on the one hand–and, on the other hand, suffering persecutory fantasies concerning the thought that if only the biological parents knew the extent of the adoptive parents' failures with the children they trusted to their care, they would despise them.[1] Pivnick (2010) writes interestingly that some adoptive parents have adopted in order to create a family in line with their wishes and dreams, to have a child of a certain gender or appearance, for instance. For those families (and children) a paradigmatic story of beneficent parental gesture to a person of inferior status rings hollow, at best. Indeed, one can argue that in these cases adoptive parents have become the new disadvantaged, with adoptees conferring status on the parents by being available for care (ibid., p. 6). But even when this is the case, the phantom object of the biological parent haunts the adoptive parent, or at least is present in the background in a way that is hard to ignore.

Finally, adoptive parents and adopted children both must deal with another phantom object: the phantom object of all the other potential adoptive parents who could have adopted this child. These transparent objects, too, are negotiated, consciously or not, in the theatre of ghosts that is the adoptive home. "Ghosts in the nursery" (Fraiberg, 1976) are a well-known phenomenon. But where it concerns the adoptive child's nursery, they are especially numerous.

Pivnick (2010) writes, justifiably, about the need for unique narratives, which rather than looking at the phenomenon of adoption through one lens, recognize its diversity and richness. The present chapter constitutes a unique, personal narrative, on the one hand, but on the other hand, as unique narratives do–it also touches a certain universal dimension related to children dealing with early traumas of abandonment and loss.

When the Actual Object Turns Away

The orphanage in which my son spent the first year of his life wasn't one of the worst. In documentaries about Romanian or Bulgarian orphanages one can see babies lying on their backs for days, never being approached by anyone, so radically immersed in their renunciation that they won't even move their hand to chase away the flies that walk over their faces.

The institution in which my son stayed took relatively good care of the infants' health and hygiene. Still, thirty babies were accommodated in one space, looked after by a rotating team of carers. To avoid outbreaks of disease, the babies were not allowed out, and so my son spent the first year of his life in one room, never exposed to daylight. The babies were fed while facing away from their carers so that neither side would form any attachment (assuming, mistakenly, that this was for their mutual benefit). This practice resulted in a mechanical disruption between the physical act of feeding and the sense of psychic nourishment that accompanies it under regular circumstances. The babies seemed to have received the food they required, but the assembly-line method whereby a baby would be fed by one carer, washed by another, then moved onto a changing table where yet another, third carer would dress them, turned the sequence of physical actions that make up primary care–which serves as an early template for communication and attachment–into a meaningless, staccato, and emotionally flat chain of actions.

In addition, since they were instructed not to communicate with the babies, carers only talked with each other over the infants' heads. The primary environment was therefore deeply inscribed with a sense of "turning-away". This turning away was not only related to the fact that these were babies that had been abandoned by their biological parents, i.e., whose first experience of their primary object was the latter's turning away from them– but also to the fact that a baby who receives no direct visual or vocal feedback when being fed and cared for will only experience relationships as a kind of turning-away. I will return to this later.

When I first met the baby I was about to adopt, motherhood was not an unknown territory: I was already the biological mother of a five-year-old son. But the baby whom the orphanage director put into my arms the moment I entered her office looked very different from the photographs that were sent to me a month or two earlier. This was not simply due to the fact that infants at this stage of life naturally change very fast. It also involved the inevitable gap between looking at a two-dimensional image and the encounter with a flesh-and-blood, three-dimensional child, something which all at once exposed–over and beyond our mutual strangeness– the arbitrariness of the "match" between us.

The gap between my first encounter with my eldest son, the child that had grown inside me, and my first encounter with the new baby who was put into my arms from the outside, was huge. For the boys' father, however, meeting the new baby was quite natural. In hindsight, I realized that the gap he had to straddle was not so significant as the one I faced: in a sense, our first son, too, had been handed to him "from the outside", and thus, the difference in directionality was much less enormous for him than it was for me. For me it was the opposite route: while my eldest son was born from inside out, my youngest son had to be born from the outside in.

I never thought adopting a child to be a one-off decision made one way or another. It was a point in time within a long process of negotiations. I don't mean the sort of negotiating with the adoption authorities or with other members of the family who were as such connected for the good and the bad. I mean negotiating with the actual possibility of relating to what may appear as pure chance—a child whom another woman has brought into the world, under conditions I will never know, wherein the sole reason for our coming together happened to be that the date of his birth coincided with the date of my application for adoption—as being in effect inevitable, that is to say, as fated.

Negotiations included all sorts of signs and portents: for instance, the fact that the name given to my youngest son when he was born was inexplicably identical to the name I'd given to my oldest son. Or the fact that the name of the city where he was born and on which my foot never trod, appeared, beyond comprehension, in a poem I'd written a year before I started to consider adopting a child. Such signs dissolved the scent of randomness that had enveloped the act of adoption. They signaled to me—or had I signaled to myself through them?—that what had seemed pure chance was in fact fated to be: this child was destined to be mine, even if in a circuitous manner whose hidden sense I would never be able to follow.

For one major source of anguish involved in adopting a child is connected precisely to this: the moment in which fate is removed from the initial pact—which is to say, the knowledge that this child could not have been born to other than these parents is nullified—the parental script turns from a riddle with a single solution into a draft that can be rewritten at any given moment. What if I had submitted my application a month earlier, or a month later? What if the first photograph of an infant presented to me had been that of the infant adopted by our close friends, and who over the years appeared in my eyes to resemble our older son far more than the infant we adopted?

I've often wondered, for example, whether it hadn't been better if a family of Sephardic origins had adopted my son: his skin tanned easily whenever exposed to the sun and turned a lovely shade of copper, completely different from the reddish skin tone of my oldest son when he remained outdoors for any stretch of time. He liked spicy food and often teased me over the Polish seasoning that went into the dishes I prepared. The TV sitcoms he loved most were always those that featured large and warm families, the sort in which one felt included on the strength of kinship itself.

During other difficult moments I thought to myself that if only he'd been adopted, for instance, by a woman whose character had been similar to my mother's, who ran our childhood home, at least at first glance, highhandedly and strictly by the rulebook–he'd have felt more secure than in the free and easy surroundings that we nurtured.

Be that as it may–and in sharp contrast to giving birth, wherein fate is in-built and sets the undertaking in motion–chance is the name of the game when proceeding to adopt a child. Hence the great mission called upon the partners in such an undertaking is to turn chance into the foreordained, a bond that bears within it an ineluctable quality that isn't inherently in-built.

The face in the first photo sent to us by the orphanage where he'd been taken in since his birth bore a worried look. He gazed sideways rather than directly at the camera, as though desperately seeking out to fix his eyes on a familiar face. He was held in the arms of an elderly woman in a blue cloak who appeared to be one of the caretakers, but she was looking at the cameraman rather than at the infant, as she exhibited him, her arms outstretched, as though holding an object whose worth she was asking the viewers to evaluate.

A month later the first video recording arrived. He looked bigger than in the first photograph, roughly five months old, and was held in the arms of the same person in a blue cloak who we now knew wasn't an attendant but rather the orphanage physician with whom he had formed a special connection, being the only child in the institution whom she called "My child."

In this video she calls him by his name and tickles him to get him to smile at the camera. He avoids laughing, because one of the other infants in the room is crying and his gaze keeps straying toward him, as though he were begging someone to calm the other infant down so that he might finally give himself over to the attention being heaped on him. The video was sent to us with an apology for the fact that they hadn't succeeded in getting him to smile and with a promise to send another video in which he would look into the camera. From the point of view of the organization attending to the process of adoption the video had been a marketing failure since it recorded a serious and anxious-looking infant.

For me, however, watching the video was the moment when chance gave way to a sense of fatedness. This fatedness wasn't connected to his pretty face, nor to the fact, which also stood out, that he appeared to be more developed vis-à-vis the other infants, responding not only to physical contact but also to the words spoken to him, which is to say that he had developed, in spite of the privations under which he grew, the ability to understand and communicate by means of a language. It was connected to the attribute that the videoed scene had underlined in effect unknowingly, and that typified him far more than any other distinction ever since: his readiness to acknowledge someone else's pain and hunger over his own.

Being-at-Home, Homelessness, Nowhere-ness

Durban (2017) suggests that a sense of home in early infancy is achieved by way of an interaction between: (a) safe dwelling in the body-as-mother (constitution); (b) internalizing the mother-as-me (internal object space) and (c) establishing a triangular Oedipal space responsible for the capacity to move between narcissism-as-a-home and the world-as-a-home. The interplay between these elements in the construction of a home is accompanied by distinct anxieties and unconscious phantasies. Disruptions in this early process, due to deficit, internal object relations or environmental factors, might lead to severe pathologies, mindlessness, hatred, and violence. Durban makes a distinction between mental states of being-at-home, homelessness and nowhere-ness based on the corresponding levels of early development and typical anxieties. He considers being-at-home and homelessness as more developed states of object relating, allowing for some capacity for feelings of loss, mourning and longing. Nowhere-ness, however, stems from early states of anxiety-of-being, characterized by confusion between self and object, nameless grief, nameless dread, and devastation (ibid.).

Adopted children seem to experience an intense disruption between the stage of "dwelling in the body-as-mother", often already disturbed by physical and mental pressures during pregnancy, and in any case severed from what happens after birth–and the stage of "internalizing the mother-as-me". Not only does the latter occur without any continuity with the stage that precedes it, but it often follows a stage of maternal vacuum (a stay at an orphanage, for instance). Maybe this is why children who were not adopted immediately after birth move between states of "homelessness"–which requires coping with loss and mourning–and states of "nowhere-ness", implying vacant, "blank mourning" (Amir, 2020). Beebe (2004) writes about what she calls "facial mirroring", quoting an adopted patient who told her: "I feel alienated from my face. My face doesn't feel like me. [...] My adoptive mother looked at me like a stranger. I didn't feel my face looked right. I couldn't look at her and find me" (p. 12). Indeed, adopted children, especially those who were not adopted immediately after birth, may experience an unbridgeable gap between the moment of their birth and the experience of finding themselves "in the face of the other". This period, characterized by what might be called "mirroring vacuum", can be thought of as part of what creates the experience of nowhere-ness.

But is it only the child who moves between nowhere-ness, homelessness and being at home? In my experience, the adoptive parent moves between these states no less than the child. Each time the child excludes themselves from the sense of home, the parent too, as the home-giver, or the one who constitutes the home for this child, experiences a sense of being cast out and exiled. The shift, thus, is not of the child alone but marks the parent-child dyad, which moves between the ability to create mutual belonging–and a sense of disconnection, disintegration, and falling into a boundless space.

This reminds me of two landmarks in my and my son's shared biography. During the first two years following his adoption, he used to ask me, several times a day, "Do you love me?" Although I answered him positively each time, it never reassured him for long, and an hour or two later he would ask me again: "Do you love me?" One day I heard him say from the other room: "You love me!" The question mark had changed into an exclamation mark. A parallel switch from question mark to exclamation mark happened to me, too: one day, when he was about two, I took him to the beach. We stood in the water, holding hands. Suddenly I saw that a huge jellyfish was about to attach itself to his leg. It was too late to move away. I lifted him up, and the jellyfish found its way to my leg instead. The pain was egregious. It took weeks of treatment till the sting healed. But inside me, this was a moment of great calm: the sense of homelessness and nowhere-ness made space for a profound sense of being-at-home.

Durban writes:

> Homelessness, the more explored phenomenon (see for example
> Papadopoulos, 2002), arouses depressive and paranoid-schizoid anxie-
> ties which deal with relationships: their dangers, gains and losses, while
> Nowhere-ness reflects several deeper archaic anxieties-of-being address-
> ing the very threat to existence as a bounded, differentiated entity in
> body, time, space and object. These anxieties are typical to developmen-
> tally damaged early mental states and include experiences such as: fall-
> ing forever, going to pieces, having no membrane or skin, being full of
> holes, losing orientation, having no relationship to the body, burning,
> freezing, liquefying and dissolving. These anxieties give rise to two spe-
> cial defensive constellations–crumbling down as described by Meltzer in
> his concept of 'dismantling' (1975), or hardening up, as in the case of the
> shell-type autistic child described by Tustin (1981).
>
> (2017, p. 181)

Collapse or disintegration, in many adopted children including my own,
often takes active forms of inversion: inner sensations of burning may
turn into active play with fire aimed to scorch, and stabilize through
scorching, the skin-shell. The experience of dissolving activates various
forms of tightening the sides of the container through actions such as hit-
ting against hard surfaces. Later this is often joined by anti-social activ-
ities and delinquency that artificially brace the subject against a sense of
flaccidity.

These actions of friction, scorching, head-banging, and later, the breaching of social and moral boundaries, testify to a state of "nowhere-ness"
which gets in the way of the work of mourning. The latter requires the
stable presence of an object which can be released from the domain of concrete relations to form an internal representation. When the mourned object,
however, was never present in the first place, what takes place is what I call
"blank mourning": various forms of concrete clinging in lieu of the ability
to represent. Banging one's head against the wall, much like scorching
or friction, come to achieve the fictive presence of a holding object or a
skin envelope (Bick, 1968). Rather than the representation of the absent
object, these acts serve the concrete conservation of that object by means
of friction with what allegedly stands in for its presence. Transgressive
or delinquent behavior may be perceived as serving the same purpose,

in so far as it is a form of constant friction against the boundaries of the law. This friction produces the experience of a present object, one against which the friction occurs, while the delinquent behavior enables an illusory, concrete restitution of what was taken away, in a manner that makes mourning superfluous. I will discuss these formations of blank mourning below, as typical of "hypertonic" compensations for the profound "relational hypotonia".

My son, like many children adopted mostly from the Soviet Union in those years, suffers from Fetal Alcohol Spectrum Disorder (Jacobson & Jacobson, 2002; O'Learey, 2004), a syndrome which is the result of the biological mother's excessive alcohol intake during pregnancy, affecting fetal brain development. One of the typical consequences of this syndrome is what seems a lack of moral judgment and a difficulty in internalizing social laws. But over and beyond an organic impairment of the capacity to judge, this involves a profound and early failure in the ability to mourn, as a result of which, instead of grieving for the lost object, an attempt emerges to magically create a "prosthetic object" which fills the objectal void by means of the omnipotent appropriation of the "object of the other".

Most difficult of all were the thefts. At first these were no more than the occasional, petty theft. Small change that wasn't returned, a money bill that most often I couldn't tell for sure whether it has been there in the first place. Little by little his boldness and actions grew more serious. I got to the point where I feared leaving my handbag out of my sight. I constantly suspected him, even when he hadn't done a thing. His response was always the same: remonstrating in anger, in tears, swearing upon his life, my life, his death. When caught in the act–he'd regularly fall back on the first year of his life as ammunition against anyone who stood against him, using it not only to justify the theft itself but also to point to our inability, the lucky ones born to parents who raised them, to understand what it was like to be him.

I could bear anything: the assorted substance abuses, the repeated attachments to young girls who took advantage of him and hurt him, the mood swings that took hold of him around any transition: from night to day, from inside to outside. But I couldn't bear the impervious freedom he allowed himself, the indifference, as I experienced it, in which he stripped us not only of possessions–but also of the ability to believe him. I didn't want to forgive, but nonetheless forgave, again and again. Until I understood that not only his pleas for forgiveness but also my subsequent granting of it, were null and void.

Stealing wasn't only an act of "reclaiming" something that he hadn't ever experienced as belonging to him. It was a form of exclusion of all those who surrounded him, their dispossession of the inherent, self-understood position of strength, of generosity (since the act of taking by force undermines first and foremost the act of giving voluntarily), of mercy. The deception was even more difficult than the theft. When it came to the latter it was possible, at least momentarily, to handle by means of rationalization (to understand, to reformulate). But deceit left us irrevocably contaminated.

During the darkest of days my psychic anguish took over my body. I developed repeated urinary tract infections that caused bleeding and sharp pains. I stopped drinking liquids out of fear of having to urinate. I scalded myself time and again, from pot handles, from the stream of hot water in the sink, from the oven. In two years, I underwent surgery for navel hernia, a biopsy for the thyroid gland and a breast biopsy. My thoughts kept straying toward death, not because I wanted to die but because I no longer knew how to love the life I had lived. I imagined it, death, as the shadow of a tree, as a brass bell, as a reservoir. I didn't want to return.

Many stood by my side during those days. And yet, I felt almost completely alone. A malicious and deafening wave of amassing hopelessness, of courage steadily fading away.

One morning, after I looked for him in the streets all night, he returned defeated. I remember that he laid his head on the wrought-iron table in our garden and for a long time I gazed at the broad nape of his neck that suddenly seemed to me frighteningly narrow. Birds twittered above the crowns of the trees their early morning twitters, and a great darkness descended over us. He entreated me to lock him up, begged that I hospitalize him in a closed ward, pleaded for my life and for his. For ninety days and ninety nights I held onto him inside our home. Time moved simultaneously forward and backward: calendar time went ahead, the stubborn and ponderous time of everyday being. But the months were enumerated in reverse as well, leading him back to his infant size, releasing from the utter silence primitive gestures of grief but also of imagination, of hostility but also of innocence.

He didn't return to the world, or "left the dark for the light", nor was he "reborn". In the end he burst open–in the sense of "cleaved" or "cracked"– from within the shell of his body. Cleaving has a different texture than reawakening or giving birth. It involves a fault, a splitting, a rupture. This rupture doesn't turn into a thing of the past. It's an exposed root needing constant attention. Like bits of eggshell stuck to the head of a chick, so too the remnants of the act of rupture remained the only thing that mattered: an eternal teetering on the brink, which has no solution other than to forcefully, determinately, hang back.

Psychic Hypotonia and Hypertonia

Tami Pollak (2009) argues that the body's holes and orifices, excepting the anus, are all located on the front of the body, creating what she calls a "frontal spine". The openings along this spine face the other person's openings. The vertebrae making up this frontal spine are junctions: not just between anatomic elements of the body-container, but also between the infant and mother who is facing it. This is an encounter in which what Pollak calls a "face-to-face relationship" comes into being.

What exactly is this relationship?

While the back of the body is opaque and bony–the front side is soft and scattered with windows. This is why when we want to make contact with a baby, we position ourselves right in front of the perceptual apertures in its face, in front of the body-windows which anatomically point out and ahead. When the mother nurses the baby, she intuitively supports both these sides: she concretely, physically supports the child from behind, while simultaneously offering emotional-communicative support from the front. This results in an infantile balance between active and passive, between what is held from behind and what turns-to, engages, reaches out (ibid.).

When a mother turns her back to her baby she turns away from the infant's frontal spine, upending this equilibrium between being held and turning-to, or yearning-for, between passive and active. The most conspicuous effect of this disruption involves what I call "psychic tone".

The word *tonus* or *tone* derives from the vocabulary of physiology where muscle tone refers to the (ongoing) partial contraction of the body's musculature. Normal muscle tone supports body posture. Abnormal states of tonicity are *hypotonia*–weaker than average basic tension–and *hypertonia*–when the muscles are excessively tense. Hypotonia and hypertonia are sometimes described as, respectively, flaccidity and spasticity or rigidity, and are observed, at varying intensity, in neurological disorders.

What then would we call "psychic tone"?

Psychic tone is the partial contraction of the psyche's muscles which produces what we might call "psychic posture." This tone is essentially bound up with the object's primary manner of turning towards the infant's frontal spine. The object's very act of facing the infant prompts the infant to respond by way of "counter-intention", triggering its psychic tone. An ongoing turning-away from the infant's frontal spine, instead, undermines his or her psychic tone: rather than stimulating them to direct themselves to the object (counter-intention), this turning-away triggers an empty, hollow attunement, one that addresses itself to a nonexistent addressee. So, while the repeated experience of turning-to encourages psychic tone, a dearth of such experience leads to weakening or even vanishing of psychic tone.

Psychic tone is a type of anchoring in the other, but at the same time it involves a securing within the infantile subject itself, which is the outcome of the other's turning to him or her. From now on, this initial turning-to will come into play in any of the subject's attempts to address any object. No addressing of an object (be it a human, a conceptual or an imaginary one) is possible without psychic tone, since the very capacity to move towards already relies on, and in turn produces, psychic muscle tension.

Psychic hypotonia is a slack, flaccid ability to aim at an object, or to maintain a psychic position that allows for any turning-to as such, whether inward or outward. Manifestations of psychic hypotonia resemble blank (Green, 1996) or pre-objectal (Kristeva, 1987) depression. Kristeva suggests that work with narcissistic patients reveals a type of depression unlike the neurotic depression resulting from ambivalent feelings toward the lost object. This pre-objectal narcissistic depression (see Chapter 1) takes a much more silent and passive form. It involves a grief that does not imply unconscious hostility toward a lost other. Rather, this is a grief originating in an incomplete, empty self. At stake here is not the loss of a whole object but of something more primitive, which rather resembles the loss of Winnicott's (1974) environment-mother. The loss, in this case, is of something, not of someone. It has been registered before the subject was even "someone", before, that is, he or she themselves amounted to a whole subject. It would therefore be more accurate to say that this is not about a loss but about a primary absence, unnamable, unrepresented, too primitive to be linked to any definite object or loss.

Psychic hypotonia is associated with the internalized presence of an object that turns away since the latter attacks precisely the ability to direct oneself to, to turn-toward, to develop a psychic tone that allows to take hold of an object. The vacant, hollow aspect of psychic hypotonia, therefore, relates to the subject's inability to turn to either themselves or the other, or in fact, to the way in which turning-away takes the place of turning-to, and undermines it.

As a defense against the great helplessness characterizing psychic hypotonia, a phenomenon of psychic hypertonia occurs. Here, turning-to the object becomes adhesive (Meltzer, 1974). In this situation the object is not recognized and met as separate and distinct, and thus, turning-to becomes a one-dimensional clinging, resulting in friction with the object's surface instead of a dialogue with its interior. For many years my son couldn't fall asleep if his foot or hand didn't touch another person's external surface. He needed the sense of concrete continuity between his body and another living body to feel that falling asleep did not mean falling forever. One such evening, he must have been about four, he said to me: "I am attached to you like the thorn to its rose."

We usually encounter psychic hypotonia and hypertonia in the form of distinct opposing tendencies. In the case of several adopted children I have met, there seems to be a combination of both, namely a combination of adhesive clinging resulting from a desperate need for friction, along with a kind of vacant flaccidity, an infinite void which not even the "adhesive" object itself can fill.

This combination of psychic hyper–and hypotonia results in a pseudo psychic three-dimensionality in which there appears to be a movement between a state of connection and a state of separation, while in fact there is a negation of both: since psychic hypotonia is not a state of separation but of non-connection, whereas psychic hypertonia is not a state of connection but rather a state of adhesion which erases both the subject and the object to which the subject clings–both hypertonia and hypotonia constitute an attack on bonding and linking. (Bion, 1959). It can be said that hypotonia is the negative of separation, while hypertonia is the negative of connection. In both cases there is no possibility of maintaining a stable mental posture, nor a stable orientation toward an other.

This deceptive oscillation between psychic hypotonia and hypertonia is often deposited in the adoptive parent as well. If the child's psychic hypotonia is manifest in a loose grip on the other as well as on him or herself–parental psychic hypotonia will be expressed in the parent's recurring urge to give up and let go. And just as psychic hypertonia develops in the child as a defense against hypotonic laxity, so too does the parent sometimes develop defensive psychic hypertonia which takes the form of over-protectiveness, vexing involvement, and efforts to control with a persecutory, compulsive quality.

How to turn this pseudo three dimensionality into a psychic space?

On Hospitality

Jacques Derrida (2000) coined the term "Hostipitality" which combines "hospitality", a word of a troubled Latin origin, with "hostility"–its very contradiction that is incorporated into it. Hospitality, in its Derridean sense, is always a radical one: it means the ability to bring in what ultimately excludes us from the position of hosts. One can think, in Derrida's terms, of adoption as radical form of hospitality, one that challenges the limits of the host's mind and body, but also allows, through this challenging, to truly let both the strange and the stranger in.

In the parental work with traumatized adopted children, the crucial task is the task of reversing the turning away to turning to, thus enabling the psychic tonus to develop and strengthen. The only way to allow this reversal is to agree to host the raw traumatic materials in an unmediated way, regressing, one may say, to the mother's primary hospitality of the fetus in her bodily container, holding it simultaneously as a stranger as well as the most welcome guest, and more than that–holding herself on the one hand as the most stable container, and on the other hand as the most flexible one, whose limits are ready to change irreversibly.

When I previously wrote about the function of the inner witness (Amir, 2012, 2014, 2019) I pointed to the infantile dependent state as what developmentally stimulates the infant's need to deviate from this total helplessness into being able to observe it and extract meaning from it. This deviation occurs through the infant's ability to turn from the initial dyad to a third–concrete or imagined–that allows them to witness themselves by means of the vantage point it provides. The importance of the inner witness is related to the ability to transform excesses. The only way to transform excesses of any kind (pain, loss, anxiety) is to create a vantage point in relation to it: to turn the nameless dread (Bion, 1962) into one that has a name and meaning.

Donnel Stern (2022) explores the formulation of experience, which depends upon the metamorphosis of experience from *not-me* to *feels-like-me,* suggesting that the movement from *not-me* to *feels-like-me* happens when we not only know or feel something, but also, and simultaneously, sense *ourselves* in the midst of this process—that is, when we know and feel that it is we who are doing the knowing and feeling. Pivnick (2013) writes about the possibility of adoptees and their families to move from feeling "lost in translation" to feeling "found in relation" (p. 60). This transition from *not-me* to *feels-like-me,* or from being lost in translation to feeling found in relation is related to the willingness of the other for radical hospitality: when the adoptive parent is ready to challenge the limits of his or her body and mind, and instead of accepting the child into a pre-prepared space–to recreate the hosting space itself–the child also learns to create him-or-herself as a vivid container.

For my son, this shift from the state of *not-me* to the state of *feels-like-me,* in Stern's words, was embodied in two unique gestures, both of which, at least to a certain degree, were addressed to me: one was his insistence on unique language disruptions, which testified to both his inherent foreignness and uniqueness, preventing their erasure; the other was his capacity to dream.

The Little Dreamer

When he began to speak, I was filled with delight: at last, he is speaking in my own tongue. But he adopted, in his great wisdom, a distorted speech. He seemed to deliberately err in the use of the singular and plural, jumbling declensions and conjugations. At first, I foolishly corrected, over and again, his mistakes. I tried to domicile him in my own tongue, as though his capacity to belong to me was dependent on it. He refused to be corrected. To himself he would repeatedly jumble up the rules of grammar, creating endless loops of errors upon errors until I relented, since I understood that correcting his speech had a far more destructive effect in terms of his capacity to belong than what I experienced as defective. And yet, I experienced it as defective. It was as if making mistakes in the language that was so precious to me made me slowdown in the face of his sharp turning away from me. Only in time did I grasp that what I understood as a turning away was in effect a turning toward me. That he turned toward me in such a fashion, by making constant mistakes, in order to establish between us what I'd sought to exclude from our common ground: the foreignness that no common language has the power to erase.

Into his dreams–from which early on he'd startle awake terrorized, often a dozen times in one night–there penetrated a strange amalgam of past and present memories: he is trapped inside the TV screen, which I unsuspectingly switch off; he is flushed into the toilet bowl; he is held in my arms as my face suddenly turns into a monster, a fiend, a witch.

Other dreams occurred alongside such nightmares, saturated with grief. When my mother died, he dreamt that upon arriving at my parents' home she greets him as always. "We haven't gotten together for such a long time," she tells him, "How come?" And he remains silent for he doesn't want to expose her to the fact of her death.

The passage from life to death, from presence to absence, was entrusted into his small hands from seemingly forever. In light of what he'd gone through he knew what the adults around him refused to know, and hence he knew what he knew in its naked and murky rawness, without their consoling mediation.

The notion of "Before its time" was connected both to his early and mature experiences. Everything was before its time, simply because his development had been reversed: death preceded life, absence preceded any form of presence.

Dreams were thus his way to reverse the direction. For as a dreamer he dreamt flawlessly. His dreams were void of shadows and bereft of secrets. They set themselves in place before him–but also before me, since he was in the habit of recounting them to me every morning–as what exists out of our reach, which precisely for that reason struck roots in us. Shards of the quotidian seemed, alongside of such dreams, as bleak lights on distant hills. They couldn't blur what the dreams themselves lit up from one end to another: the unassailable mystery of abandonment.

But dreaming also saved him. With the blinking of an eye upon waking, his wide-open lids seized in part the overlapping ends of the inner and outer, an overlaying that formed an indissoluble bond between the two worlds.

In this way minute bits of daylight penetrated the gloom of night. The blue door of the toy closet cast from time-to-time sheaves of color on the closed lid of the coffin in which he was locked. The sun-drenched windowsill, on which there sat a happy row of furry dolls, naturally extended the railroad tracks anticipating the train that threatened to run over him. Alongside the worried look on his face there appeared in time flickering moments of inexplicable joy, which were possibly connected with the simple fact that the days began and ended without his being dropped; that the catastrophic severance dividing the time of the birth of the body and the time of the birth of the soul was stitched back together, at least to a degree, by means of the thread woven between sleep and wakefulness.

I never loved him more than I loved him when he woke from a dream: for a brief moment, partially baked in his sleep's thick webs, he let me, too, bridge the act of abandonment with that of salvation (since for him, not knowing any other mother, I had always been both: the mother who deserted him and the mother who gathered him unto her bosom); the sin alongside the atonement of sin (for the sin of abandonment, from the moment it becomes a possibility, is the possible sin of all mothers); the fact of life, related to his actual coming into the world, with the spirit of life, which is what could only be given to him by the power of my love.

Note

1 Of course, the birth parent who gave a child away could also experience this actual child as a phantom object.

References

Amir, D. (2012). The inner witness. *International Journal of Psycho-Analysis*, 93, 879–896.

Amir, D. (2014). *Cleft Tongue: The Language of Psychic Structures*. New-York and London: Karnac Books.

Amir, D. (2016). When language meets the traumatic lacuna: The metaphoric, the metonymic and the psychotic modes of testimony. *Psychoanalytic Inquiry*, 36(8), 620–632.

Amir, D. (2019). *Bearing Witness to the Witness: A Psychoanalytic Perspective on Four Modes of Traumatic Testimony*. London & New-York: Routledge.

Amir, D. (2020). The bereaved survivor: Trauma survivors and blank mourning. *Psychoanalytic Perspectives*, 17(1), 74–83.

Beebe, B. (2004). Faces in relation: A case study. *Psychoanalytic Dialogues*, 14(1), 1–51.

Bick, E. (1968). The experience of the skin in early object-relations. *International Journal of Psycho-Analysis*, 49, 484–486.

Bion, W. (1959). Attacks on linking. *International Journal of Psycho-Analysis*, 40, 308–315.

Bion, W.R. (1962). A theory of thinking. In: *Seconds Thoughts* (1967). New York: Aronson, pp. 110–119.

Deeg, C.F. (1989). On the adoptee's cathexis of the lost object. *Psychoanalysis and Psychotherapy*, 6, 152–161.

Derrida, J. (2000). *Of Hospitality* (trans: Rachel Bowlby). California: Stanford University Press.

Durban, J. (2017). Home, homelessness and nowhere-ness in early infancy. *Journal of Child Psychotherapy*, 43(2), 175–191.

Fraiberg, S. with Adelson, E. and Shapiro, V. (1976). Ghosts in the nursery. *Journal of the American Academy of Child Psychiatry*, XIV, 1975. *The Psychoanalytic Quarterly*, 45, 651.

Green, A. (1996). The analyst, symbolization, and absence in the analytic setting. In: *On Private Madness*. London: Routledge.

Jacobson, J.L., and Jacobson, S.W. (2002). Effects of prenatal alcohol exposure on child development. *Alcohol Research & Health*, 26, 282–286.

Kristeva, J. (1987). *Black Sun: Depression and Melancholia* (trans: Leon S. Roudiez). New-York: Columbia University Press.

Meltzer, D. (1974). Adhesive identification. In A. Hahn (ed.), *Sincerity and Other Works: Collected Papers of Donald Meltzer*. London: Karnac Books.

Meltzer, D., Bremner, J., Hoxter, S., Weddell, D. and Wittenberg, L. (1975). *Explorations in Autism: A Psycho-Analytical Study*. Strath Tay: Clunie Press.

O'Learey, C.M. (2004). Foetal alcohol syndrome: diagnosis, epidemiology and developmental outcomes. *Journal of Paediatrics and Child Health*, 40, 2–7.

Papadopoulos, R.K. (ed.) (2002) *Therapeutic Care for Refugees: No Place Like Home*. London: Karnac Books.

Pivnick, B. (2010). Left without a word: learning rhythms rhymes and reasons in adoption. *Psychoanalytic Inquiry*, 30(1), 3–24.

Pivnick, B. (2013). Being borne: Contextualizing loss in adoption. *Psychoanalytic Perspectives*, 10(1), 42–64.

Pollak, T. (2009). 'The "body-container": A new perspective on the "body-ego"'. *International Journal of Psycho-Analysis*, 90(3), 487–506. http://dx.doi.org/10.1111/ijp.2009.90.issue-3

Quinodoz, D. (1996). An adopted analysand's transference of a 'hole-object'. *International Journal of Psychoanalysis*, 77, 323–336.

Rosenberg, E. (1992). *The Adoption Life Cycle: The Children and Their Families Through the Years*. New-York: The Free Press.

Rosenberg, E.B., and Horner, T.H. (1991). Birth parents romances and identity formation in adopted children. *American Journal of Orthopsychiatry*, 61, 70–77.

Sopher, R. (2018). An allegiance to absence: Fidelity to the internal void. *Psychoanalytic Quarterly*, 87(4), 729–751.

Stern, D.B. (2022). On coming into possession of oneself: Witnessing and the formulation of experience. *Psychoanalytic Quarterly*, 91, 639–667.

Tustin, F. (1981). *Autistic States in Children*. London and Boston, MA: Routledge.

Winnicott, D.W. (1974). Fear of breakdown. *International Review of Psychoanalysis*, 1, 103–107.

Chapter 6

On Forgiveness

Years ago, when my son was about four, I went to pick him up from kindergarten and found him with his back turned to his best friend and the teacher, at her wits end, between them. They just had a fight, and the kindergarten teacher couldn't convince either one of them to ask the other to forgive him. It was late. The other boy's mother was furious, and it was time to lock the building. What to do? I proposed that instead of asking for forgiveness, they might offer forgiveness. Each of them could tell the other: "I forgive you". After offering forgiveness, it might be easier to ask for it. And so it was.

What is this ability to forgive?

For years I have been witnessing the way in which internalized objects and their real-life derivatives, or conversely, real-life objects and their internalized reverberations, travel all the way to the underworld and back in order to allow for a healing which is usually too little, too late. What occupied me while writing the present chapter was the capacity for reparation, not merely in relation to concrete damage but also as an inner point of departure.

The groundwork of forgiveness, like that of regret, is a priori, as I understand it, at least to some degree: it is present as a potential, prior to the deed to be either regretted or forgiven. This echoes, in a way, Klein's ideas in "Envy and Gratitude" (1975 [1957]) concerning the ability to constitute a good object. According to Klein, this ability is not merely the outcome of the presence of a good external object which the child internalizes. It is also the very condition for turning an object into a good one, in the sense that the child needs to have an a priori ability to recognize and internalize good objects as such, a groundwork of goodness, a structural ability for gratitude.

In her "Mourning and its Relation to Manic Depressive States" (1940), Klein describes herself (who in the article appears as Mrs. A.) walking in

DOI: 10.4324/9781032715766-6

the street not long after the death of her young son, when the beauty of the surrounding buildings strikes her: "Her relief at looking at pleasant houses was due to the setting in of some hope that she could recreate her son as well as her parents; life started again in herself and in the outer world" (p. 111).

A little before that she writes:

> Mrs. A., who in an earlier stage of her mourning had to some extent felt that her loss was inflicted on her by revengeful parents, could now, in phantasy, experience the sympathy of these parents (dead long since), their desire to support and to help her. She felt that they also suffered a severe loss and shared her grief, as they would have done had they lived.
>
> (p. 110)

When catastrophe befalls us, it also befalls our inner objects (Roth, 2020). Mrs. A. (Klein herself) is angry at her inner parents who did not protect her from the catastrophe, but also feels guilty towards them, because this catastrophe happened to them inside her as well, reviving her guilt over all the pains they experienced in the past and are now going through due to the current loss. Her tears testify not only to her painful recognition of her loss, but also to the good and strong connection with both her lost object and her inner objects–a connection of love that gives comfort in the face of pain and sorrow (ibid.).

Klein's description offers a unique portrayal of the process of reparation. She releases her internal objects from the omnipotence she attributed to them when she blamed them for her catastrophe. Now she can be in touch with the damage this catastrophe has left in those internal objects as well, who endure both the loss and their inability to save her from it.

The capacity to extract her internal objects from their omnipotence is, for her, the real reparation. Not the restoration of their omnipotence, that is, their returning to the status of her saviors–but rather the renunciation of this omnipotence, and through this renunciation the regaining of the ability to be in touch with what they can still give her. Klein describes the moment when she realizes that although they are not the cause of her disaster, and cannot save her from it either, they mourn her loss together with her, inside her, and it is this ability to experience them as sharing her mourning that allows her to feel that she can join them in shared sorrow: "The tears that she shed were to some extent the tears that her internal parents shed, and she also wanted to comfort them as they–in her phantasy–comforted her" (Klein, 1994 [1940], p. 110).

Amihud Gilead, in his book *Saving Possibilities* (1999), makes a distinction between the mentally "possible" and the physically "actual". Since the actual is also possible, but not everything that is possible is also actual–the possible is a broader category than the actual and includes and encompasses it (Gilead, 1999, 2003). In my book *On the Lyricism of the Mind* (Amir, 2016a) I suggested a different distinction between the mentally possible and the mentally actual, or between the "possible self" and the "actual self"–a distinction which rather than being situated in the body-mind dimension, as Gilead proposed, obtains exclusively in the domain of the psyche. I suggested to consider the "actual self" as the actualized part of mental life (whether conscious or unconscious), and the "possible self" as the part which resides in the mind as an unrealized yet present psychic possibility. Between a person's birth (the transition from possible to actual) and a person's death (the passage from actual to possible), a whole life spans, consisting of a reciprocal and continuous motion between the possible and the actual. Whenever a contact between a person's actual self and their possible self occurs–the possible undergoes actualization in the sense of becoming manifest as a part of that person's mental life. However, the possible that does not become fully actualized also exists throughout in the form of inner lining, or an additional dimension, endowing the actual existence with depth and resonance. The lyrical dimension of the mind, which is, as I suggested, a type of integration between the actual self and the possible self, is the mechanism that enables the subject to stray from their concrete biography by means of this motion back and forth between contact with the actual and contact with the possible.

But contact with the possible is not a merely internal event: it is an important component of our interaction with others as well. One fascinating manifestation of this can be seen in some children, who develop, for reasons which are partly constitutional, a sufficiently strong lyrical dimension, and as a result manage, in the course of object internalization, to make contact with the object's possible qualities rather than with its merely actual ones. In that way, for instance, the child of a sick and depressed mother might be able to register her possible love and care for him through the actual wall of maternal dysfunction. Or a child of a violent father would be able to make contact with the warmth that never found actual expression but nevertheless existed as a possibility. However, the opposite direction is also relevant: a child of a gentle and tender father may perceive the father's possible aggressiveness, just as a child of a warm and caring mother may feel her possible melancholic tendency beyond her actual excellent functioning. The presence of this imaginative, "lyrical" dimension, so I assumed, enables us to be in touch with what is beyond the actual constraints of our objects, allowing us to transcend not only their actual biography but also our own. Our capacity to tolerate both the other's shortcomings and faults, as well as our own, is related, at least to some extent, to the capacity to be in touch with a "possible" unbroken layer, in both self and other, which allows a transcendence of the concrete present and movement toward a more comprehensive perception of both self and object.

When contact with this layer is not possible, what occurs is a collapse into the concrete realm of the actual object or the actual self. Contact with the object's unbroken possible is then replaced by the image of the omnipotent object. The difference, however small it may appear, between the unbroken possible object and the omnipotent object, is critical: making contact with the possible layer already involves the work of mourning over what has never become actual, and this mourning also includes an experience of the object mourning what it did not manage to actualize or give. Contact with the object's omnipotent image, by contrast, implies a refusal of the work of mourning: in the case of such a refusal, the object is perceived as having chosen to deprive the child from what is theirs by right, and keep it to itself. The object then is perceived as envious and triggers a similar envy. Contact with the object's possible layer is therefore also what enables forgiveness, because it is associated with the assumption that the object could regret what it was unable to either be or give. Adherence to the object's omnipotence, by contrast, because it assumes the object's refusal to regret, involves the subject's refusal to forgive. *There is, in other words, a profound connection between the subject's ability to see the object as capable of regret and the subject's ability to perceive it as deserving forgiveness.*

Three Positions on the Axes of Self and Other

I would like to offer a kind of mapping, referring to the relation between the subject's perceiving of the object as capable of regret and the subject's capacity for forgiveness. This mapping marks three positions, from malignant to benign, located on the respective axes of object and subject.

The most malignant position on the axis of the object is the position of *evil* or *indifference toward evil*. In this position, the object—in the subject's perception— wishes to inflict pain or alternatively is indifferent to the other's pain. The object in this position is experienced as able to feel neither guilt nor regret. On the axis of the subject, this position is paralleled by a position of vengefulness, which seeks to repeat the original injustice, as Hannah Arendt (2018 [1958]) has suggested, only with reversed roles. When the subject thinks of the object as having evil intentions toward him or her or as being indifferent to the evil that befalls them, the subject will develop a fantasy of vengeance in which he or she aims to inflict on the other what the other (or its representations) has inflicted on them.

The second position on the axis of the object is the position of *guilt/atonement*: feelings of guilt that lead to attempts at atonement. I have previously discussed acts of atonement, especially in regard to collective victimizers (Amir, 2017, 2019; Amir & Hacohen, 2020). Gestures of compensation and appeasement where one nation has committed an injustice against another have been on record throughout history. One instance was when Germany committed itself to make reparation payments to Holocaust survivors worldwide. Another instance was the Peace and Reconciliation Committees set up by South Africa's postapartheid government, aiming to compensate and rehabilitate those who suffered under the regime. I put these two very different examples side by side to bring out the difference between *atonement* and *regret* (the object's third position, which I will describe shortly). While the disguised aim of atonement, as I perceive it, is to cleanse the abuser and to erase or undo the act of injustice, regret connotes a recognition of the injustice and its implication for the other, which is only then followed by an effort to repair. While atonement constitutes an act that seeks to undo what happened by means of compensation, regret opens a new space. This distinction between acts of atonement and gestures of regret may cast light on some Holocaust survivors' refusal to accept German restitution payments, which they experienced as a type of erasure of the injustice rather than a recognition of its meaning and implications. The Peace and Reconciliation Committees, by contrast, were seen by those who took part in the process as aiming to recognize, rather than erase, the injustice.

On the axis of the subject, the parallel of the position of guilt/atonement is the position of *amnesty*, which is located between the position of vengeance and the position of forgiveness. While this position does not repeat the original violation, like the position of vengefulness, it does not escape the symmetry of inversed power relations either. On the contrary: the gesture of amnesty is squarely situated within power relations. The one who grants amnesty occupies a position of power in relation to the other and so remains locked in the existing power relations, if not by way of malignant inversion of power (like in the position of vengeance), then by way of reaction-formation. In this intermediate state, the one who grants amnesty takes hold over the other through this very act, exempting that other from punishment—but not from guilt (Amir, 2022).

The third and final position on the axis of the object is the position of *regret*, which has its parallel on the subject axis in the position of *forgiveness*. These two positions, regret and forgiveness, share, much more than the two other pairs, a dimension of mutuality. We can think of the object who is capable of regret as enabling, by dint of that regret, the subject's transformation into someone who can forgive. But at the same time, and not less importantly, we can think of the subject's ability to forgive as what makes it possible for the object to feel regret. Regret, thus, is the outcome of forgiveness no less than what prompts it.

Though these three positions seem clearly demarcated, in most cases there is a dynamic movement between them, and so we may assume that they are present, with fluctuating dominance, in any encounter, whether concrete or imagined, between subject and object.

Between No Regret and No Forgiveness: "Something Disguised as Love"

In her memoir *Something Disguised as Love* (2021; Hebrew), Galia Oz unfolds a succession of abuses to which her father, the Israeli writer Amos Oz, subjected her throughout her childhood. The memoir takes the shape of an indictment composed, in addition to her own testimony, of quotations from the psychological literature (functioning as "expert opinions"), things reported by childhood friends, and accessory evidence deriving more or less directly from letters her father wrote to her.

The memoir's main addressee is not the father but the witnesses, or jurors, who are summoned, throughout the book's chapters, to pass sentence on him. This is the memoir's strength but also its weakness. Rather than entering a conversation with its audience, it demands that they pass judgment. Over and beyond not holding out any possibility of amnesty, it seems to constitute a public execution.

In terms of two-dimensional versus three-dimensional perceptions of the object, one might say that the more layered and multivocal the representation of an object, the less exposed it is to reduction, thus evoking a more ambivalent and stratified response. Respectively, the more the object's three-dimensionality flattens, approaching two-dimensionality, our judgment, too, becomes flattened. The memoir's flattening of the father is not accidental. This is an intentional act, even if not necessarily conscious, one that serves to guide the reader's thought toward one particular place. As Oz writes near the end of the memoir: "This is a test for the readers too, especially those who doubt" (p. 135).[1] In addition to its flattening of the father, the text does the same to its readers, removing any possibility for them to think differently from what the writer requires them to think. The result is a "hermetic" narrative (Amir, 2016b), where the grave in which the narrator feels she was buried alive transforms into a hermetic text that obscures any possible living dialogue or thought.

"Each outburst enfolded an entire morality-spectacle," she writes, "starting with the crime (mess, rudeness, and sometimes nothing whatsoever), followed by holy rage and resounding punishment, and finally expulsion" (Oz, 2021, p. 29). It is hard not to observe how the text itself enacts this entire spectacle all over again, while achieving a perfect role reversal: enumeration of the father's crimes, rage (holy, or at least accompanied with an aura of absolute justice), removal, banishment, and, finally, now that the memoir is published, resounding punishment.

"This mental abuse, which is everywhere, resembles a huge octopus sending its tentacles in all directions", writes Oz (ibid., p. 30). Her memoir, too, sends its tentacles everywhere, outflanking the reader wherever possible. Whenever readerly doubt might slip in, the text inserts evidence, quotes experts, and shifts into generalizations and the plural. Since the father is never perceived as being capable of regret, even when he makes gestures an outsider might understand as such, pardon or clemency are out of the question, let alone forgiveness.

When a different picture emerges for a moment, it is immediately placed within walls that prevent it from "leaking," in the minds of the readers as well as in the mind of the writer, into the other pictures:

From early childhood I frame one picture marked by peace and quiet: a rainy, stormy night. I am a toddler in rubber wellies and my father and I are on our way to the children's home, chatting under the umbrella while above our heads enormous casuarina trees shake their branches like in a whirlwind.

(Ibid., p. 33)

The need to isolate and "frame" this picture as a singular one is typical of the hermetic narrative exemplified so clearly by this text: the slightest leakage of one memory into another, of good into bad, puts the entire structure at risk of crashing. This is because it relies entirely on exclusion, on separation between one element and another, on a polarization that rules out any possibility of the integration of different qualities.

Traumatic memories have the tendency to barricade and isolate themselves from all other memories. As a result, living aspects of the self cannot flow toward them or form an associative link with them. Because of the fear that the new memories may become "infected" with the traumatic ones (and vice versa— the fear that the traumatic memories will be mixed with everyday materials), the psyche may end up creating a hermetic wall that prevents access to the traumatic memories. In that way, they continue to dwell within the mind as facts, but it is extremely difficult to create a vivid movement to or from them and to transform them by means of such a movement from solid to flexible psychic matter (Amir, 2016b). This isolation puts the traumatic narrative into a kind of psychic formalin jar that preserves it as a coherent sequence at the cost of retaining its static and frozen state. A "pseudo-access" to the traumatic contents thus takes shape: on the one hand, as we see here, the testimonial narrative is kept tight and convincing. On the other hand, this convincing narrative has a double role: it simultaneously preserves the story while withholding any transformative access to it. This also explains the refusal of any attempt to inquire, to observe from a different angle, or to question the absoluteness of memory. This refusal casts the reader in the role of a captive audience convened for the purpose of passively validating the narrative, a muted audience, of which the narrative effectively demands that it erase itself as a subject and become, instead, an object in the service of the story (Amir, 2016b).

This is the core connection between the hermetic narrative and the mechanism of identification with the aggressor (Ferenczi, 1933). In fact, it can be understood as a variant of the primary traumatic event itself: the victim, who was forced, at least in her experience, to surrender her subjectivity and become a hostage in the service of her father's needs, becomes herself the one who, by means of her testimonial narrative, now forces her listeners or readers to surrender as thinking subjects, turning them into passive extras in a spectacle in which they otherwise take no part.

Still, Oz's narrative includes a few moments of a different quality as well. One such moment begins as follows:

> What is it about this scene, a quiet, free morning in a tidy home where making noise is forbidden, Cantata number 106 playing in the background at a low volume—that even now makes me feel despondent, so many years after that home stopped to exist? Why does this clean picture hound me?
>
> (p. 34)

I myself wondered, while reading, why it was here that my eyes teared up. It was not the description of the father's deploring of any music other than the type he preferred; neither was it the picture of the daughter's small hand reaching out quickly for the gramophone's arm to avoid scratching the record. The memoir is full of far more grating images than this one. The effect of this moment is related to its formulation, which, for a brief moment, moved from statement to question. This question opened a door in me as well, allowing me, as its addressee, to soften for a moment in the face of this tightly frozen narrative and enter the picture, rather than watch it merely from outside.

At some point, Galia Oz introduces the notion of "gaslighting,"[2] which she defines as "a manipulation which is aimed to unsettle a person by means of the constant questioning of his testimony, his judgment, his sense of reality, and even his sanity" (ibid., p. 59). This phenomenon is particularly interesting here. There is no question about the existence of this mechanism, which operates especially often in the case of abusive families, but also in various political settings. But in the present instance, it is fascinating to observe how the same notion may also apply to the memoir itself, which, like hermetic narratives in general, creates its own conditions of truth, thereby making it impossible to question them.

In a letter in which "he confesses his guilt," the father writes: "'You were slapped a few times. You were sent out of the house a few times. You were cold–shouldered,'" but, she adds, "He removes himself by using an impersonal construction. Who sent me away and turned their backs? [...] The confession undermined itself, cunningly denied itself" (p. 62).

Here the reason for the inability to absolve, let alone forgive, becomes clear. The father's admission is perceived as shrewdly undermining itself. Not only is it not experienced as the outcome of regret, but it is felt like a cynical manipulation, typical of perpetrators' language (Amir, 2017), in which their actions are worded in the third person instead of the first person in order to disguise their responsibility for them. The same happens in the following passage:

> *You're always right,* he wrote, *maybe a little too right. Only once in thirty or forty years did you ask me to forgive you.* I tried to read this sentence and avoid resisting, be open to the possibility that I too had to repair some historic injustice I committed against him. I was willing to ask for his forgiveness, but nowhere were there any details of the sins for which I was responsible. And then, at another point in his letter, I realized the nature of my original sin: *You loved me more than daughters should love their father* (in these very words, exactly).
>
> (Ibid., p. 63)

When I described earlier the inability to release the object from its omnipotence, I had in mind precisely what these lines convey. In addressing his daughter with these words, the father seems to be saying something about the omnipotent proportions to which she, out of her childish need, inflated him, and that it is these huge proportions that now make her unable to forgive him.[3] The issue of this omnipotence returns when an excellent anonymous review of one of Galia Oz's children's books turns out to have been written by her father. Here, as well, he presents himself (and is perceived by her) as omnipotent: someone who not only is able to bring off this "fraud" but also takes pleasure in the frustration it causes:

> He clearly delighted in my frustration, the plot he wove against me, the superiority he derived from leaving me in the dark. [...] This was not done in innocence but as an obsessive attempt to get a grip, once more, on what he thought was his and had escaped him.
>
> (Ibid., pp. 67–68)

In 2018, she recounts, he phoned her for the last time:

> During that conversation, I wasn't aware that this was the last time we
> were talking. I was impatient and tense. The sound of my father's voice
> scared me. If only he would have let go of the ambiguity, if only he had
> just managed to utter one expression of goodwill, said one thing that was
> sincere. I expected him to say he loved us, that he missed us after all this
> time, and so on. None of that happened. [...] I am trying to find a way
> to come to my father's defense, span a bridge over the abyss which time
> and his death have opened up between us. Maybe he did try to admit his
> mistake but didn't manage it because of his fear of humiliating himself.
> But no, he was a tough dealer who showed no sign of empathy. [...] He
> neither expressed regret nor promised to repair.
>
> (Ibid., p. 96)

There's a momentary attempt here, from her side, to build a bridge: to see
him or conceive of him as capable of feeling sorry even if he is unable to
express it. But the effort collapses in view of her experience of him as cal-
culated and manipulative:

> He never showed a sign of being troubled by his conscience, he only
> demonstrated the distress of someone who has been forced to defend
> himself against the powers of darkness. He was wretched because of
> what I forced him to inflict on me.
>
> (Ibid., p. 105)

Here we get to what I see as the crux of this memoir:

> The friends I am talking about [friends who like her were slapped or
> otherwise abused in their childhood–DA] are able to love their vio-
> lent parents due to a certain quality these parents had and which, in the
> absence of a common Hebrew expression, I would call compassion [...].
> Compassion, in this loose definition, is the very essence of parental feel-
> ing. [...] It is something that enfolds a child at every single moment, a
> transparent layer yet very concrete, which constrains but also ensures a
> kind of decency, even in the harshest of homes.
>
> (Ibid., pp. 113–114)

Galia Oz sees her father not only as someone who does evil, but also as being complacent about it. His sin is twofold: if only, like other violent fathers, he would regret what he did or acknowledge its severity, even while justifying doing these things for educational reasons, for example, she could have felt compassion and maybe even forgive. But the hostility she describes, the hostility she experienced, is a "transparent hostility." As a result of (and as a defense against) this transparency, Galia Oz's narrative takes on a double function: in the face of the transparent hostility, it erects a hermetic, high-security barricade that encircles what lacks in outline, paints the colorless, and transforms what has slipped out of view into something that fills the field of vision entirely. This is its power. But this fortification also has the effect of locking the very act of writing and thinking within its boundaries. The result is that the text fails to create dynamic or vital movement. It is, rather, a carefully planned track whose start and end have been determined in advance and that constitutes execution of judgment rather than any process of revealing.

Amnesty as Inversed Power Relations: "Letter to the Father"

"Letter to the Father" (1953) is a letter Franz Kafka wrote to his father that never reached its destination. Kafka presents in this personal text an entire spectrum of father-son relations in order to map the ways in which his father oppressed and suppressed his son's capacity to make his stand or even fully become himself.

The letter opens with the reason for its writing:

> You asked me recently why I maintain that I am afraid of you. As usual, I was unable to think of any answer to your question, partly for the very reason that I am afraid of you, and partly because the explanation of the grounds for this fear would mean going into far more details than I could even approximately keep in mind while talking.

> (ibid., p. 3)

This opening already sets the tone for what is about to follow: The father's question, at least as the son remembers it, is not "why *are you* afraid of me?" but rather "why *do you maintain* that you are afraid of me?" (ibid.). The question already weakens its addressee: maybe you don't really have a reason to be afraid of me but just convince yourself, or me, that you are?

The letter then goes into a detailed description of the various dimensions of the father's omnipotence, beginning with a comparison between the father's body and the son's ("There was I, skinny, weakly, slight; you strong, tall, broad. Even inside the hut I felt a miserable specimen, and what's more, not only in your eyes but in the eyes of the whole world, for you were for me the measure of all things"; p. 7) and continuing with the father's way of violently imposing his views ("You had worked your way so far up by your own energies alone, and as a result you had unbounded confidence in your opinion. [...] Your opinion was correct, every other was mad [...] and finally nobody was left except yourself"; p. 8) and with the manner in which he disapproved, outright, and without having made their acquaintance, anyone in whom the son showed the slightest interest ("It was enough that I should take a little interest in a person [...]—for you, without any consideration for my feelings or respect for my judgement, to move in with abuse, defamation, and denigration." p. 9).

The father's very size or proportions make him, in the eyes of his son, unforgivable. The primary violence (Aulagnier, 2001) resulting from the physical differences in size and power, even without turning into actual violence, excludes the child from the father as well as from himself. Along the pages of this long letter, the son sums up his father's sins against him, including acts he interprets as violent even though they were meant generously, and moments when the father seemingly turned to him to help. The father, as the son perceives him, thinks only of himself, and even when he seems to turn to the boy, he in fact turns his back on him or takes the opportunity to humiliate him. So, for instance, when the young man tells his parents about his sexual experiences, taking the opportunity to let them know that because they left him "uninstructed," he exposed himself to great dangers. The father's response is to tell the son that he can help him "go into these things without danger" (p. 32)—which may appear a caring and open-minded response if only the son wasn't so preoccupied with issues of power:

What you advised me to do was in your opinion and even more in my opinion at that time, the filthiest thing possible. That you wanted to see to it that I should not bring any of the physical filth home with me was unimportant, for you were only protecting yourself, your house. The important thing was rather that you yourself remained outside your own advice, a married man, a pure man, above such things; [...] Thus you became still purer, rose still higher. The thought that you might have given yourself similar advice before your marriage was to me utterly unthinkable. So there was hardly any smudge of earthy filth on you at all. And it was you who pushed me down into this filth–just as though I were predestined to it with a few frank words. And so, if the world only consisted of me and you (a notion I was much inclined to have), then this purity of the world came to an end with you and, by virtue of your advice, the filth began with me.

(ibid.)

I dwell on this paragraph because here, maybe more than anywhere else in this indictment, the son's blind spot in relation to himself is most striking. The accusation is clear: under the cover of giving his son good advice, the father installs the hierarchy between them according to which he, the father, places himself above anything filthy (here in the form of sexuality), while instead pushing his son right into it. The son sets aside the fact that it was he who informed his parents of the risks he had apparently taken and blamed them for not instructing him back then, and in addition, he assumes (or maybe projects) that the father, before his marriage, never indulged in things he now urges his son to partake in. It seems that no matter what advice the father would have offered his son, it would have been understood in the same way. Had the father, for example, reprimanded him for engaging in these sexual practices, it would have been understood as affirming the hierarchy just as much as when he responded how he actually had, in a relatively open-minded, nonjudgmental way.

This leads to what in many ways could be taken as the text's crux:

Sometimes I imagine the map of the world spread out and you stretched diagonally across it. And I feel as if I could consider living only in those regions that either are not covered by you or are not within your reach. And, in keeping with the conception I have of your magnitude, these are not many and not very comforting regions [...].

(pp. 41–42)

The son is unable to live except for in the regions that are not covered by the father's body—but even those sparse regions are covered with the father's shadow, something that makes them uninhabitable for the son. This, by the way, is what the son himself says further on when commenting on his father's advice:

> Here perhaps both our guiltlessness becomes most evident. A gives B a piece of advice that is frank, in keeping with his attitude to life, not very lovely but still, even today perfectly usual in the city, a piece of advice that might prevent damage to health. This piece of advice is for B morally not very invigorating–but why should he not be able to work his way out of it, and repair the damage in the course of the years? Besides, he does not even have to take the advice; and there is no reason why the advice itself should cause B's whole future world to come tumbling down. And yet something of this kind does happen, but only for the very reason that A is you and B is myself.
>
> (Ibid., pp. 32–33)

This letter, then, is not written from just one perspective. It is scattered with evidence of another position, one that, in terms of the present essay, we might call the position of amnesty. Here, for instance, is evidence of this position:

> And in saying this I would all the time beg of you not to forget that I never, and even for a single moment believe any guilt to be on your side. The effect you had on me was the effect you could not help having.
>
> (p. 5)

While the son does not forgive his father at these moments, he is willing to absolve him. In this imaginary act of granting his father amnesty, the son simultaneously enacts the roles of prosecutor, witness, judge, and executor. In doing so he does not release himself from the power relations between himself and his father but rather inverts them so that he now absolves his father from his superior position as a judge. This reversal culminates at the end of the letter, where the son replies to himself in his father's name and goes one step further by also replying to his father's imagined reply. The confusion the son creates when addressing himself in the father's voice, then replying to the imagined version of the father and even going along to argue with some of the arguments put forth (by himself), points exactly at what is so necessary in order for forgiveness to be possible: at least some separation between father and son, some ability to conceive of the father as a subject in his own right who exists beyond his alleged overshadowing of his son, and equally the perception of the son (by himself) as a subject in his own right who exists over and beyond the shadow of his father.

The son responds to himself on behalf of the father, staging a play in which the father allegedly speaks as a subject, with a voice of his own. But in fact, this subject does not really speak in the voice of the father but in the voice of the son imagining the voice of the father. The son's voicing (or ventriloquizing) of the father is in fact a silencing of the latter and an inversion of the perceived power relations: now the father is the one who is silenced, while the son both addresses himself in the father's voice and answers in his own, removing the father from the entire conversation exactly by means of arrogating the power to give him a voice. What we witness here is the way in which in granting amnesty, as opposed to forgiveness, the power relations, fundamentally unquestioned, are simply inverted. While forgiveness offers room to the other, granting amnesty is an act of eliding the other exactly under the guise of offering him or her a space.

Forgiveness as Refusing a Pact with the Devil: "Satan Says"

Sharon Olds' poem "Satan Says" (2017)[4] does not mention forgiveness even once. Its negotiation is between the speaker, locked in a little cedar box, and Satan. Satan comes to her in the locked box and says, *"I'll get you out. Say /My father is a shit."* When she repeats after him Satan laughs and says: *"It's opening. /Say your mother is a pimp."* Again, she repeats after him. Something "opens and breaks" when she says that. The way out is through Satan's language, that is, through her joining of his language. This is the code that opens the lock. And indeed, every time she repeats after him, something opens a little, but not only opens. Something also breaks. The verb "break" appears twice in this poem. The second time appears in the following lines: *"Say shit, say death, say fuck the father,* /Satan says, down my ear. /The pain of the locked past buzzes /in the child's box on her bureau [...]./ Shit. Death. Fuck the father./ Something opens. Satan says /Don't you feel a lot better? /*Light seems to break on the delicate /edelweiss pin, carved in two /colors of wood." And so, we understand that there is a price to pay for opening this box. Something will break. It is virtually impossible to open without breaking something irreparably. Here appears her first gesture of resistance to the covenant with Satan: "I love him too, /you know, / I say to Satan dark / in the locked box."

I would like to linger, for a moment, on the word "too," which makes the very transformation in this poem. The speaker does not erase the past, nor does she annihilate the child's buzzing memories. And yet, by using the word "too" she deviates from the flat dichotomy of love-hate. It is possible to hate and love the same person, even at the same time. "Satan softly says, *Come out./* But the air around the opening/ is heavy and thick as hot smoke./*Come in,* he says, and I feel his voice/ breathing from the opening./ The exit is through Satan's mouth./*Come in my mouth,* he says, *you're there/ already,* and the huge hinge/ begins to close./ Oh no, I loved/ them, too, I brace/ my body tight/ in the cedar house." The covenant with Satan makes it possible to get out only in one way, through his mouth, that is, through the one idiom he offers. But in the first lines of this poem the speaker says: "I am trying to write my/way out of the closed box". She tries to "write her way out," that is, to find, through her own words, a path out of the place in which she is imprisoned. However, to come in Satan's mouth is not to write *her* way out but rather to write *his* way in. What seems a possibly orgasmic rescue is nothing but a repeat of what locked her in the cedar box in the first place. And to that she refuses by saying– "Oh no, I loved/them, too".

What happens at this point of refusal? The speaker counters the language Satan offers—a language that by repetition of the words aims to repeat the torture— with a different language: "I loved them/ too." In the face of the radical polarization held out by Satan, the "too" she extends resurrects the three-dimensional image of relations in all its complexity. These three-dimensionality and complexity are, as the rest of the poem shows, the spell that expels Satan, who "sucks himself out the keyhole", leaving her locked in the box, sealing the heart-shaped lock with the wax of his tongue.

"It's your coffin now, Satan says./ I hardly hear;/ I am warming my cold/ hands at the dancer's/ ruby eye—/ the fire, the suddenly discovered know-ledge of love."

As far as Satan is concerned, she buries herself alive at this very moment. If she is not ready to "only hate," she has no way out. But for her, the gained knowledge of love has a much greater power to free her than the old knowledge of hatred. Against Satan's tongue, which seals the heart-shaped lock with its wax, leaving her inside, there is another fire, perhaps another tongue, which might melt the wax and open the box in a different way, "suddenly discovered," unthought-of before. And so, there is a lyrical reversal here that transcends the rules that the poem sets, violating the covenant with Satan's language in favor of the covenant with a language of her own. Instead of coming "in his mouth," on his terms, she comes in her own mouth, with her own words, on her own terms. Unlike Galia Oz and Kafka in their letters to their fathers, Olds neither seeks revenge nor pretends to grant amnesty. Her journey is a journey inward, not one that leads her toward an actual other. Her goal, unlike that of the two others, is not situated externally (confession, recognition) but aims to attain another inner state. It is a voyage of forgiveness exactly because rather than turning away from the thing that must be forgiven, it allows her to turn toward it in her own language.

The Departure Point of Forgiveness

In an essay "On Forgiveness", dedicated to the relations between Hannah Arendt and Martin Heidegger, Michal Ben-Naftali writes:

> Arendt believes that only forgiveness, which has the effect of reversing what has been done in the past, can redeem the public space from the irreversible nature of our actions, freeing us from their consequences instead of leaving us trapped in them. Only forgiveness can allow us to start anew for a common future. Forgiveness is therefore contrary to revenge, which for Arendt means a re-execution of the original offense–an act that does not put an end to the first act but leaves all parties bound within it. [...]. Revenge is a natural and automatic response to an offense. You can expect it. You can even calculate it. Forgiveness, however, is unpredictable. It is not conditioned by what aroused it, and it has the power to unshackle both the one who forgives and the one who is forgiven. [...] Arendt's forgiveness is a demonstration of freedom. The freedom to choose who you want to be. The freedom to transcend.
>
> (2019, pp. 129–130)

Unconditional forgiveness of this kind, which transcends the conditions that led to its very occurrence, is not an act that hallows the perpetrator's behavior; rather, it puts itself over and beyond it.

In his book *The Gift of Death*, Jacques Derrida (1996) claims that true forgiveness consists in forgiving the unforgivable. Were forgiveness granted only to the forgivable, then the very idea of forgiveness would disappear. In other words, an act that is forgivable does not require forgiveness. Forgiveness is always radical forgiveness. It is only required or becomes meaningful where forgiveness is impossible. It is neither an economic event of give-and-take nor does it require any specific conditions (for instance, the violator asking forgiveness) in order to be achieved. Forgiveness is the opposite of all this: it is outside the language of negotiation and hence unnegotiable.

I would like to take the idea of forgiving the unforgivable as a point of departure, but also challenge it, or suggest expanding it, with the notion of *a spectrum of forgiveness*. On this spectrum, there also exists forgiveness for what *can* be forgiven, even if not without difficulty. This kind of forgiveness is situated on the axis I described before, higher than amnesty, because it is an act of liberation, of freedom, for the one who forgives just as much as for the one who is forgiven, and because it institutes, as suggested earlier, a reciprocity, a bidirectionality, with regret.

The forgiveness for the unforgivable is of a different order and requires a different positionality. It is not a specific act but a broader attitude, one I would call a departure point of forgiveness. From this perspective, forgiveness is not a response to something that has already happened, but a preexisting possibility. Derrida claims it is a mistake to think that forgiveness, which is already attributed to a vertical movement, is always sought from the bottom up or is always granted from the top down. But the departure point of forgiveness, as I see it, doesn't only reverse directions but erases the hierarchical movement in itself: it removes power from the giver and weakness from the taker, thereby entirely undoing the "economic" relations of giving and taking, turning forgiveness from being a transitive action to an intransitive state.

A key text illustrating this departure point of forgiveness is the diary of Etty Hillesum, a twenty-seven-year-old woman, written in Amsterdam between 1941 and 1943.

[…] I knew at once: I shall have to pray for this German soldier. Out of all those uniforms one has been given a face now. There will be other faces, too, in which we shall be able to read something we understand:

that German soldiers suffer as well. There are no frontiers between suffering people, and we must pray for them all.

(1996, p. 156)

This is just one of many instances of Hillesum's attitude throughout the
pages of her diary. The position she presents refuses the power relations of
victim and victimizer to which she is prompted by rejecting what Ferenczi
(1933) called "the terror of the sufferers," which victims' suffering imposes
on their surroundings. Her refusal of the victim position is not based on the
denial of suffering but rather feeds from a transformation of the victim-
victimizer dichotomy into a notion of human responsibility in which those
located in both sides equally participate.

The departure point of forgiveness ties together forgiveness and responsibility. The ability to forgive is a way of taking responsibility for self and
other or, rather, for the human and the humane, which both self and other,
victimizer and victim, embody in different variations, even if from opposing sides. This type of responsibility can be blurred both by the position of
the helpless victim and that of the guilty victimizer.

Hillesum's diary is full of illustrations of this responsibility:

There is a really deep well inside me. And in it dwells God. Sometimes I
am there, too. But more often stones and grit block the well, and God is
buried beneath. Then He must be dug out again.

(Ibid., p. 44)

Or elsewhere: "And God is not accountable to us for the senseless harm we
cause one another. We are accountable to him!" (Ibid., p. 150).

Merav Roth (2020) writes:

Hillesum does not manically exclude herself from the human fate. Her
strength lies in her courage not to split and project onto people, and to
avoid the urge to create a world of external bad objects and internal good
ones. Instead, she has a profound understanding that in each person,
including herself, good and bad reside, and that the choice of the good
is by no means obvious, but is an option in every conceivable situation.

(Ibid., p. 543)

Does this amount to saying that there is nothing that cannot be forgiven?
Clearly not. Nor does it imply that it is incumbent upon each and every one

of us to attain this point of departure of forgiveness in the face of the unforgivable, whatever it may be. The array that stretches between the forgivable and the unforgivable is a personal one, and in addition to being personal, it may be conceived of as a line along which one may move, taking different positions over the course of life (or the course of therapy), even in relation to the same event or object. We have the option, in other words, to take a more complex position than between a dichotomous forgiveness versus nonforgiveness. And this ability to create a continuum on which we shift among different positions at different points in time in itself releases us from the fixity of nonforgiveness with a welcome stirring of life.

Forgiveness is not only a choice. It is our most profound way of taking responsibility for ourselves and for others, and this means that, however difficult this is to recognize, we have a certain responsibility for the suffering the other has caused us as well. This must not be understood as the masochism of turning the other cheek, nor is it some confirmation of what is known as "victim guilt". The point here is rather that being part of humanity, no one of us has immunity: neither from being on the receiving end of evil, nor from being its agent. "Suffering has always been with us, does it really matter in what form it comes?" writes Hillesum (1996, p. 152). The forgivable, for her, is not a singular action or person, but *humanity as such*, over and beyond its singular manifestations in individuals and their deeds. In terms of the departure point of forgiveness, we forgive not because the other's deeds *deserve forgiveness*. We forgive because the ability to forgive is the only antibody with which the human spirit can counter the unforgivable itself.

Notes

1 This and the following quotations were translated from the Hebrew original by Mirjam Meerschwam Hadar. There is currently no published English version.
2 A term deriving from George Cukor's 1944 film *Gaslight*.
3 Not to mention that this particular father was already inflated because of his huge success and fame.
4 Sharon Olds, "Satan Says" from *Satan Says*. Copyright © 1980 by Sharon Olds. All rights are controlled by the University of Pittsburgh Press, Pittsburgh, PA 15260. Used by permission of the University of Pittsburgh Press. Source: *Satan Says* (University of Pittsburgh Press, 1980).

References

Amir, D. (2016a). *On the Lyricism of the Mind: Psychoanalysis and Literature.* New–York: Routledge.

Amir, D. (2016b). Hermetic narratives and false analysis: A unique variant of the mechanism of identification with the aggressor. *Psychoanalytic Review*, 103(4), 539–549.

Amir, D. (2017). 'Screen confessions': A fresh analysis of Nazi perpetrators' 'new-speak'. *Psychoanalysis, Culture & Society*, 23(1), 97–114.

Amir, D. (2019). The last of the unjust: Test case of a screen confession. *International Journal of Psychoanalysis*, 101(3), 597–610.

Amir, D. (2022). On revenge, pardon and forgiveness. *Journal of the American Psychoanalytic Association*, 70(6), 1111–1135.

Amir, D., & Hacohen, N. (2020). Screen confessions: The test case of 'Breaking the Silence'. International *Journal of Applied Psychoanalysis*, 17(4), 296–312.

Arendt, H. (2018 [1958]). *The Human Condition.* Chicago: University of Chicago Press.

Aulagnier, P. (2001). *The Violence of Interpretation* (trans: Alan Sheridan). London: Routledge.

Ben-Naftali, M. (2019). *Towards a Minor Autobiography.* Jerusalem: Carmel.

Derrida, J. (1996). *The Gift of Death* (trans: David Wills). Chicago: University of Chicago Press.

Ferenczi, S. (1933). Confusion of tongues between adults and the child. In M. Balint (ed.), *Final Contributions to the Problems and Methods of Psychoanalysis.* London: Karnac Books, pp. 156–167.

Gilead, A. (1999). *Saving Possibilities: A Study in Philosophical Psychology.* Amsterdam: Rodopi.

Gilead, A. (2003). How does love make the ugly beautiful? *Philosophy and Literature*, 27(2), 436–443.

Hillesum, E. (1996). *An Interrupted Life and Letters from Westerbork.* New York: Holt Paperbacks.

Kafka, F. (1953). *Letter to the Father* (trans: Ernst Kaiser, Eithne Wilkins). New-York: Schocken Books.

Klein, M. (1975 [1957]). Envy and gratitude. In *Envy and Gratitude and Other Works 1946–1963.* New-York: The Free Press, pp. 176–235.

Klein, M. (1994 [1940]). Mourning and its relation to manic–depressive states. In Rita V. Frankiel (ed.), *Essential Papers on Object Loss.* New-York: New-York University Press, pp. 95–122.

Oz, G. (2021). *Something Disguised as Love.* Modi'in: Kineret Zmora Bitan, Dvir.

Roth, M. (2020). Mutual witnessing between a writer and her readers in Etty Hillesum's diaries, 1941–1943. *Psychoanalytic Review*, 107(6), 531–549.

Index

For Product Safety Concerns and Information please contact our EU
representative GPSR@taylorandfrancis.com Taylor & Francis Verlag GmbH,
Kaufingerstraße 24, 80331 München, Germany

Printed and bound by CPI Group (UK) Ltd, Croydon, CR0 4YY
08/06/2025
01897008-0017